YOGA
FOR ADDICTION RECOVERY

8 LIMBS, 10 BODIES, 12 STEPS

PATTY (PATWANT) WILDASINN

Companion soundtrack by Jap Dharam Rose
Illustrations by Israel Ron
Edited by Dr. Dorothy Wills
Cover by Dr. Mandi Batalo

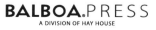
BALBOA.PRESS
A DIVISION OF HAY HOUSE

Balboa Press books may be ordered through booksellers or by contacting:

Balboa Press
A Division of Hay House
1663 Liberty Drive
Bloomington, IN 47403
www.balboapress.com
844-682-1282

Because of the dynamic nature of the Internet, any web addresses or links contained in
this book may have changed since publication and may no longer be valid. The views
expressed in this work are solely those of the author and do not necessarily reflect the views
of the publisher, and the publisher hereby disclaims any responsibility for them.

The author of this book does not dispense medical advice or prescribe the use of any technique as a form of
treatment for physical, emotional, or medical problems without the advice of a physician, either directly or
indirectly. The intent of the author is only to offer information of a general nature to help you in your quest
for emotional and spiritual well-being. In the event you use any of the information in this book for yourself,
which is your constitutional right, the author and the publisher assume no responsibility for your actions.

The exercises and recipes in this book come from the teachings of yoga. No medical advice is intended
or given herein. Always check with your personal physician or licensed health care practitioner before
making any significant changes in your lifestyle or exercise regimen to ensure that any changes may
be appropriate for your personal health condition and for any medications you may be taking.

Interior Image Credit: Israel Ron

ISBN: 979-8-7652-3311-5 (sc)
ISBN: 979-8-7652-3312-2 (e)

Library of Congress Control Number: 2022915116

Print information available on the last page.

Balboa Press rev. date: 08/25/2022

Contents

Acknowledgements

The task of acknowledging everyone who contributed to the creation of this book feels overwhelming. The list spans a lifetime. I acknowledge and give credit to all of the individuals who helped to make me who I am today. It's the relationships in recovery, yoga, and beyond that gave birth to this project. My gratitude is immense.

I would like to give special thanks to those who shared their creative hand in this project; editor Dr. Dorothy Wills, illustrator Israel Ron, cover design Dr. Mandi Batalo, the many who shared personal testimonials, and especially to Jap Dharam Rose for recording the very beautiful and functional companion soundtrack.

Preface

Where did this come from?

This entire book on 12 Step recovery and yoga was originally going to be a single chapter in my first book, *Yogable, A Gentle Approach to Yoga for Special Populations.* As I began to dive into writing on this topic, I quickly saw that there was just too much information to share in one chapter. As I was contemplating simply deleting the chapter on addiction and dealing with it later, I had an *Akashic Record Reading* that confirmed this was the right decision. In the most rudimentary sense, the *Akashic Record* stores all information of current and past incarnations on a cosmic level. An analogy would be similar to how the grooves on a vinyl record contain the music notes, lyrics, and songs. The facilitator told me that I would be writing a whole book on yoga and addiction in the next five years. The timing is about spot on.

Both addiction and yoga are topics near and dear to me, and I realized personal insight into the workings of recovery and yoga would be beneficial in book form. I have attended yoga trainings with wonderful information about using yogic technology to support addiction recovery. The teachers have had intellectual knowledge, but have lacked personal experience with addiction. Don't get me wrong, I'm not passing judgement, they have helped many people, but I understand why they are left baffled and in tears when someone they are trying to help leaves yoga and returns to using behaviors and drugs of choice. Addicts have an amazing ability to be manipulative and enchanting. Addiction is an affliction of deep self-centeredness. Both the 12 Step programs and yoga derive from spiritual principles and encourage connection with a like-minded community, which helps to relieve the obsession of self.

It is not my intention to outline the 12 Steps in their totality, or tell people how to work a program. My goal is to provide insight into addiction and recovery through the use of the 12 Steps and yoga, sharing a technology of body and breath, as well as the mind. I intend to introduce the concepts of yoga that support the entire recovery process, and I will share helpful practices that can be used in a concrete and practical way.

The 12 Step programs are anonymous in nature, and so right off the bat I stretch beyond my comfort zone in a very public way. As a recovering addict I have maintained my anonymity in both private and public sectors of my life, and have been reticent in sharing on the level of full self-disclosure. When my children were young, it was a choice made on their behalf as well as my own. That time is over now, and I am very openly breaking my anonymity in the hope of helping others. If just one person reads something that helps them stay in recovery one more day, move more deeply into a relationship with self or a Higher Power, or try a practice that makes them feel good, then my goal is accomplished.

Some of the basic yoga information shared within these pages comes from my first book, *Yogable.* It is shared in a condensed manner in order to prepare for the yoga experience outlined for each of the 12 Steps.

May you approach these pages with an open mind and willing attitude. This book is put together in a way that it may be used by individuals seeking a personal practice, or for yoga teachers wanting to teach those in recovery, possibly in treatment centers, prisons, sober living centers, or private yoga studios. Adapt the information to your own personal needs and/or target audience.

1

What is Addiction?

I was almost dead from my addiction by the time I was twenty. Physically still alive, but spiritually and emotionally bankrupt, I was hopeless and full of despair. I hated everyone, but most of all I hated myself.

As far back into childhood as I can remember, I felt as though I didn't quite belong. I felt uncomfortable in my own skin, insecure, angry and fearful, although I knew not why. I felt like I missed the secret to life. On the outside it sure appeared to me like others knew something I did not.

My first intentional experience with alcohol, at the age of fourteen, filled the dark void within. The alcohol filled the empty hole. Even though I ended the night with my head in the toilet, I was in love. I found the solution to my internal dis-ease and couldn't wait to drink again. I had found liquid comfort and courage. I made a conscious decision that night that I was going to drink when I grew up.

It was on! The disease of addiction did not wait for me to grow up; it took over immediately. The use of chemicals was an attempt to soothe internal conflict, although I would not have been able to make that identification in the early stages of using. I was drinking and experimenting with substances as often as I could, and very shortly after I turned seventeen, I was shooting heroin. I was after total obliteration through silent, self-destructive rebellion. At first, the drug culture lifestyle was actually quite fun. It took me out of my self and eased self-doubt. My engagement with life was aloof at best, as the drugs ran through my veins in a desperate attempt to fill the inner void. The punk rock music scene echoed the rebellious attitude in my mind. I'm sure I often smelled like stale beer and a smoky bar, even though I wasn't technically old enough to be in one. Ahh, the 1980's in Los Angeles and Hollywood.

In a short period of time my life became a blur. What initially worked to numb, and offer an escape from reality, quickly turned dark and out of control. As tolerance increased, I could never get enough.

I recall having moments of clarity, but was unable to stop using of my own volition. I tried a geographic move by going out of state to college, punk rock rebel turned sorority girl.

PATTY (PATWANT) WILDASINN

I should note, I had excellent chameleon skills back in the day. It was there I remember waking up one morning out of money (which was the norm), wondering with desperation where I was going to get a drink that day. I was only nineteen years old and had a glimpse of clarity where I knew that this was no way to live, that maybe I had a problem. After all, I only went to school to get out of living in a tent trailer with my friend in her sister's backyard. That was actually a pretty sweet deal, comparatively speaking, but I couldn't stay in that tent forever. The glimpse of clarity faded and I left school after one year, still intoxicated. Moments of clarity would revisit, but left to my own devices I was unable to change, or do anything different. A sinking feeling of reality crept in one night when I found myself shooting drugs with water out of a puddle at a gas station. In an attempt to not inject gasoline, my friend and I decided we should taste the puddle water first. I remember putting that disgusting, brown water in my mouth and thinking I could not believe where life had taken me. How did I end up here? However, as soon as the needle hit home it temporarily did not matter.

The cycle of addiction is vicious. As I was caught in this cycle at such a young age, I did not have much to lose, and what little I did have in the way of self-respect and self-esteem, I freely gave away. For many people this process takes longer and includes the loss of family, home, jobs, finances, and maybe incarceration, but I quickly hit the curb. I had a job waiting tables that was not as secure as I'd believed, and I could barely keep gas in the tank of my car. My family was baffled by my behavior, and I isolated from them as much as possible. I always thought I would kick dope next week and then things would get better. I even believed it over and over again. I learned later that repeating the same behavior over and over expecting different results is the definition of insanity. Living in active addiction is insanity. It is a self-imposed prison.

Before I was able to move out of this prison, I had to admit complete defeat. By the time I got to this place of total powerlessness I saw no way out, and had no intention of living beyond the age of thirty. I could not seem to muster any change on my own, no matter how miserable I was with my life.

So, at twenty years old I was worn out, sick, and apathetic. When I was unexpectedly confronted by my family, my heart spoke instead of my head and I asked for help. This surprised the hell out of me. I believe asking for help was a form of Divine Intervention because that's not what was going through my head. Evidently, I was in enough pain to be honest. I had to leave everything behind.

Now, I made choices in my addiction to be practically indigent, but that's not how I was raised. I ended up hospitalized in Beverly Hills with lobster brunches and a whole host of detox drugs.

After ten days, I was whisked away to a residential rehab facility. I stayed in residence for one year, beginning an amazing journey of 12 Step recovery and a life beyond my wildest dreams. I assure you many days in that first year I stayed simply because I had nowhere else to go.

I was quickly plugged into the 12 Step fellowships. I have found the steps to be an essential and integral part of living clean and sober, profound personal growth, accountability, and responsibility. It is only through taking responsibility that we can have freedom.

I also learned that the inner void was something I could not fill on my own. No amounts of drugs or alcohol, cookies or cigarettes, would actually fill the hole; it was a connection to spirit that was needed. An honest plea to an unknown Source began an awakening to the self.

I was about a dozen years into recovery, and had been working as a chemical dependency counselor for over a decade, when I ended up in my first Kundalini yoga class. I was in a place of both gratitude and emotional pain. If you are familiar with the 12 Steps, you know that growth and change is an ongoing process, and that being stagnant can be deadly. I wasn't exactly stagnant, but I needed more. Yoga was the technology to deliver a radical change. I loved the active meditation and the yogic teachings resonated deep within my being.

I knew within six months I wanted to teach yoga and share it with the recovery community. As I learned more, practiced more, and experienced more, I began to see a correlation between the 12 Step principles and the 8 limbs of yoga that are the basis of yogic philosophy. The ideals weave together to support the realization of our full human potential and the power to create a happy and healthy life, free from active addiction. This is the message I wish to share in the pages that follow.

How is Addiction Defined?

"My life in active addiction was an unexamined matrix of disturbances held at bay by addictive behaviour. The stimulus-response relationship between me, myself and the world was like this, 'I'm lonely – have sex, I'm sad – get drunk, I'm bored – eat a cake.' It probably wasn't even that articulate." -Russell Brand (2017)

The nature of addiction, or substance use disorder, is truly pathological. It's an insidious disease that tells the addict they don't have a problem or illness, even though the evidence is contrary. If you're confused, don't worry; so was I.

An accurate and well accepted definition of addiction, adopted by the American Society of Addiction Medicine (2019), states that *"addiction is a treatable, chronic medical disease involving complex interactions among brain circuits, genetics, the environments, and an individual's life experiences. People with addiction use substances or engage in behaviors that become compulsive and often continue despite harmful consequences."* Basically, even though the addiction damages life on a physical, emotional, mental, or spiritual level, it is not enough to deter the addictive behavior and it continues. It continues even when there is a desire to stop. An incongruency in beliefs and actions causes further suffering within the addicted person.

There is not a single factor to identify as the cause of addiction. To reiterate, predisposing factors may be environmental influences, traumatic experiences, genetics, and physiology, but we also need to look at the fact that each person processes information differently. For example, I have a sister and two brothers, and out of the four of us I'm the only one in need of a 12 Step program.

"Addiction is distinguished from drug use by the lack of freedom of choice." - Gorski/Miller (1986)

As early as 1946, E.M. Jellineck, a pioneer in alcohol studies, described alcoholism as *"any use of alcoholic beverages that causes damage to the individual or to society or both."* Alcohol may be substituted with any drug of choice or addictive behavior in regard to damage caused.

The identification as an addict, the owning of the disease, is done by the individual. Family, friends, bosses, and physicians may see clearly the problem, but the individual has to own it themselves before any progress is to be made. Family members or friends cannot love or force the addict out of their addictions. Repeated attempts to control others creates its own cycle of addiction called co-dependency. There are several questionnaires in the treatment and recovery realms designed to assist one in determining if the use of chemicals or repetitive behaviors is addictive in nature. One of the main questions addicts ask is, *"How do I know if I really have a problem?".* I don't want to share multiple or complicated surveys in the pages herein, but I will share a long standing and concise four question assessment used by addiction professionals, titled CAGE. Again, substitute drinking with using drugs or any addictive behavior of choice.

CAGE Questionnaire

- *Have you ever felt you should **C**ut down on your drinking?*
- *Have people **A**nnoyed you by criticizing your drinking?*
- *Have you ever felt bad or **G**uilty about your drinking?*
- *Have you ever had a drink first thing in the morning to steady your nerves or to get rid of a hangover (**E**ye opener)?*

Scoring:

Item responses on the CAGE are scored 0 or 1, with a higher score an indication of alcohol problems. A total score of 2 or greater is considered clinically significant.

Even if findings are clinically significant, it is the admission of the individual that is important in creating change. This is a process that has to be done with honesty, and ultimately for the self. Outside pressures may introduce a person to treatment or recovery; work, family, a nudge from the judge, etc., but for recovery to be successful it must at some point transition into a personal commitment. Quite frankly, as I look at the questions above, if you have not felt bad or guilty about your using or drinking, and if no one has said a word to you about it, you may not be done. Guilt is felt as one moves through the cycle of addiction, and then it's broken down and dealt with as one moves through the stages of recovery.

We will get to the stages of recovery later in the book. Since this chapter is exploring addiction itself, it is worth noting there are also stages of dependency. Addiction does not occur as an event. The disease grows and develops, sometimes slowly and sometimes quickly, but many times beyond the conscious awareness of the addict themselves. The first stage is a growing dependency, or needing the drug or behavior to feel good. The second or middle stage of dependency is a progressive loss of control, using, eating, drinking, gambling, etc. more than planned. The addict may cross personal boundaries put in place to control the use or behavior. The third or final stage of dependency is physical, psychological or spiritual sickness. More simply stated, an inner emotional resonance of being sick and tired of being sick and tired. By the time the addict enters the final stage of dependency they are exhausted by the endless cycle.

The cycle of addiction plays out in thought, behavior and feeling. It is a cycle that spirals out of control, with limited opportunity for intervention best applied at the level of feeling between the stages of spiritual bankruptcy and obsession. The cycle of addiction is depicted as adapted by the Addiction Model by Allen D. Flock (1986).

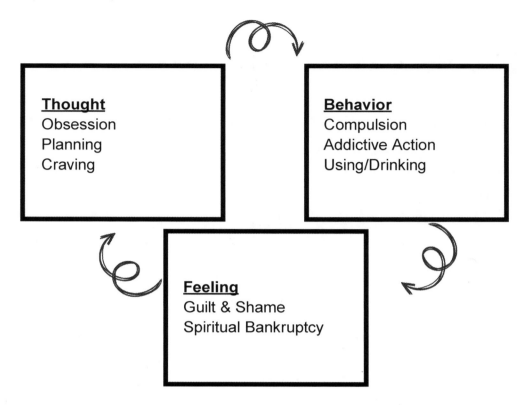

I don't care what your fixation is or what you are addicted to: cigarettes, food, alcohol, narcotics, gambling, sex, shopping, self-defeating patterns of thinking, whatever - we have a saying in the 12 Step program that *"One is too many, and a thousand is never enough."* One fix, one drink, one purchase, one donut, one bet, one in and of itself will not quell the craving, but only exacerbate it. It is akin to pouring fuel on a fire. An unlimited supply of the "one" doesn't work either because the exhaustion from continued addiction wears on the soul, and coupled with an increase in tolerance, renders what was once seen as a solution, ineffective. The drug or behavior of choice simply stops working like it once did. The disease will never satisfy itself. Recovery is a solution that takes honest, diligent work and total change. Recovery is more than abstinence.

Abstinence alone does not sustain the soul of the addict. Addiction is a sneaky, cunning disease that continues to progress. Recovery requires more than eliminating the identified substance or maladaptive behavior. Inner and outer change is necessary.

There is no quick yoga cure for addiction either. Yoga can be used for energy management, just as steps are applied for behavior management. One of the best benefits yoga can give to those in recovery is relaxation. This is especially true for those in treatment centers and new to recovery. Yoga is also helpful in supporting the recovery process because both yoga and the 12 Steps adhere to similar spiritual principles. Yoga may be thought of as solely a physical practice, especially if you're only looking at the cover of yoga magazines while in the checkout line at the grocery store, but at its core yoga is a spiritual practice. Yoga is not just something to do, it is a way of being and interacting with the living world that fits right into the 12 Step lifestyle.

"Addiction is a special kind of Hell. It takes the soul of the addict and breaks the hearts of everyone who loves them." - Addiction Angels and Answers

The disease of addiction does not have a cure based in medicine, but a reprieve and reparation based in spirituality. The addict cannot pop a pill to make the addiction go away, but through introspective healing and support, recovery is possible. Recovery is available to everyone, but it must be personally chosen and claimed.

2

Chakras

I know the title of the book mentions limbs, bodies, and steps, but I am going to begin by sharing about the chakras because they weave through the entire body and the aspects of yoga and recovery presented in this book. The chakras are like fountains of energy and provide the foundation for the expression of the 8 Limbs, 10 Bodies, and 12 Steps. So, what exactly is a chakra?

"Chakra is a Sanskrit word used by the Hindus. It literally means 'wheel of light.' Each chakra has four discernible characteristics that functionally affect the aura: color, size and shape, rotation or spin, and intensity (or amount of energy produced.) As a chakra spins, it produces its own electromagnetic field, which combines with the fields generated by the other *chakras* to produce what we call the auric field." – from *Wheels of Light* by Rosalyn L. Bruyere (1989)

"Chakra means 'wheel.' Chakras are energy centers, or energy vortices. They exist as dynamic energies, and they can help us to understand the way energy is processed by a human being within the vast and complex interplay of a multi-leveled existence. The eighth *chakra* is the aura. It appears to be an oval or a circle of light. The aura combines the effects of all the other chakras." – from *The Aquarian Teacher* (2003)

Chakras are spinning circles of energy that influence the body on a physical, emotional, mental and spiritual level. They plug us into the universe and are deeply tied to our health and well-being. Yoga typically refers to the seven main *chakras* which vibrate along the spinal column, and the aura as chakra number eight (as I will also for the purpose of this book). These centers are independent, but interconnected. Each person vibrates their own unique auric personality. The color and strength of the aura is a projection of the chakras (energy centers of the body), which in turn is a projection of the physical, emotional, and spiritual state within each person at any given moment. The aura is not static, it fluctuates.

"The Aura is our projection and protection. It catches things that may hurt us. Be they physical disease or toxins or mental attacks such as criticisms. In doing so, it can have things get stuck to it, become scratched, dented or even torn and shredded.

Keeping the Aura maintained and healthy gives us a chance to live with grace and ease. It acts as our windshield as we drive down the highway of life. A windshield catches the dirt, rain, and bugs before they get to us. You CAN drive with a dirty windshield. You'll find yourself squinting and leaning forward, straining to see the road ahead OR you can clean that windshield and find you are leaning back, relaxed and really enjoying the ride.

The Aura is the window that protects you, yet allows you and your intuition to see what's next." - Victoria Rose (2022)

A healthy aura is flexible and can extend 9 feet around the body in all directions. The primary, or inner, aura extends out around the body approximately 4-5 inches. This primary aura can be felt and experienced by anyone. Let's try a little experiment now. Rub the palms together briskly until heat is created, then bring the palms facing each other, about 6 inches apart, in front of the body. From here begin to slowly move the palms toward each other and back out, palpating for a gentle resistance. When you come up against a slight resistance, as if you're holding a bubble, this is where the edges of the primary aura meet. This will give you an idea of the size of your inner aura. Although an edge to the aura can be sensed, it does continue to subtly penetrate and interweave through the universe. The aura radiates from within the body in response to our worldly experiences.

In the yogic teachings it is said that the use of drugs and alcohol has adverse effects on the aura, creating weakness, ripples, or even holes that allow outside energies to seep into the individual energy field. This is one way dis-ease can enter into the energy field. As observed and shared by healer Rosalyn Bruyere, one shot of liquor doubles the size of the primary aura. It spreads the aura, not making more of it, but stretching the aura thin so it becomes blurry. Only one shot of liquor creates less reactive availability, with continued regular use exacerbating decreased reactivity in the energy field. Another example of how illicit substance affects the aura is the use of methamphetamine, or speed. Methamphetamine creates a crisp edge to the aura, blocking the ability to filter and process information accurately. The use of chemicals negatively affects the user beyond the physical and emotional body, permeating the individual energy field. When we carry dis-ease from addiction the chakras can become inflexible and obstructed.

Chakra Basics

First Chakra: Muladhara – The Root of Foundation

Location: Base of the spine
Color: Red. Bone marrow chi (energy) is red and regenerates during sleep.
Element: Earth
Sense: Smell
Qualities: Concept, Desire for safety, Fight or flight response, Habits
Physical: Elimination, Adrenals, Bones, Feet, Rectum, Large intestine
Unbalanced: Fear, Weak constitution, Addictive behavior, Tunnel vision, Self-centered, Feelings of not belonging, Insecurity, Desperation, Lack of control
Balanced: Secure, Loyal, Trust, Living in the moment, Valuing oneself, Self-awareness, Stability, Confidence, Feeling grounded
Yoga Postures: Crow, Chair, Frogs, Front stretches
Foods: Red apples, Beets, Pomegranates, Protein
Gemstones: Garnet, Red Tiger's Eye, Red Jasper
Aromatherapy: Lavender to stimulate, Patchouli to calm

Second Chakra: Svadhistana – Sweetness

Location: Sacral spine, about 2 inches below the navel
Color: Orange. Bone vibrates orange. Exercise builds bone, moves and clears emotion through the body.
Element: Water
Sense: Touch
Qualities: Feeling, Creativity, Empowerment, Sexuality, Desire, Relates to change and flow of life, Motion, Passion for life and hobbies, Appreciation, Joy
Physical: Kidney, Bladder, Reproductive organs
Unbalanced: Shallow relationships, Shame, Sexual irresponsibility, Guilt, Rigidity, Helplessness
Balanced: Responsible relationships, Creative, Expression of intimacy, Empathy, Sense of others, Patience, Allowing for good things
Yoga Postures: Frogs, Cobra, Butterfly, Cat-cow
Foods: Oranges, Pumpkin, Carrots, Seeds, Nuts
Gemstones: Moonstone, Carnelian, Orange Calcite
Aromatherapy: Amber to stimulate, Rosemary to calm

Third Chakra: Manipura – Lustrous Gem, Will of Spiritual Warrior

Location: Solar plexus, about 2 inches above the navel.
Color: Yellow. Yellow is a mental color and can be used for learning or studying.
Element: Fire
Sense: Sight, both physical and creative.
Qualities: Opinion, First link to life, Physical health, Personal power, Will, Logic, Reason, Assimilation, Judgement, Honor
Physical: Digestive organs, Muscles
Unbalanced: Greed, Anger, Despair, Low self-worth, What's in it for me attitude,
Balanced: Inner balance, Self-esteem, A sense of command over life, Leadership skills, Stability, Empowerment, What's in it for us attitude
Yoga Postures: Stretch Pose, Bow, Fish, Breath of Fire
Foods: Yellow peppers, Bananas, Yellow squash, Lentils
Gemstones: Citrine, Tiger's Eye, Honey Calcite
Aromatherapy: Bergamot and Ylang-Ylang to stimulate, Rose to calm

Fourth Chakra: Anahata – Unstruck

Location: Heart Center
Color: Green. The skeletal muscles vibrate green.
Element: Air
Sense: Touch
Qualities: Feeling, Expansiveness, The middle way, Compassion, Unconditional love, Kindness, Truth, Clarity, Balance, Transition, Acceptance
Physical: Heart, Thymus, Arms, Hands, Lungs
Unbalanced: Grief, Loneliness, Hurt, Attachment, Dependent, Emotionally isolated, Resistant
Balanced: Love, Harmony, Detachment, Forgiveness, Neutrality, Self-love, Service, Living in the present, Absence of judgement and expectation
Yoga Postures: Heart opening postures, Baby pose, Arm work
Foods: All leafy greens, Broccoli
Gemstones: Emerald, Jade, Green Aventurine
Aromatherapy: Pine and Honeysuckle to stimulate, Sandalwood and Rose to calm
Additional: The purpose of the heart chakra is to perpetuate love.

Fifth Chakra: Vishudda – Purification

Location: Throat
Color: Blue. The fascia (connective tissue beneath the skin) vibrates blue.
Element: Ether
Sense: Sound
Qualities: Response, Personal domain, Creative destiny, Communication, Truth, Expression, Language, Subtle connection, Integrity
Physical: Throat, Neck, Shoulders, Thyroid, Parathyroid
Unbalanced: Manipulative, Shy, Bold in speech, Expression problems, Insecurity, Frustration
Balanced: Healthy expression, Authentic, Truthful, Effective, Hear what's not been said, Consistency
Yoga Postures: Neck work, Mantra
Foods: Honey, Blueberries, Figs, Kelp
Gemstones: Aquamarine, Blue Kyanite, Blue Apatite
Aromatherapy: Patchouli to stimulate, Lavender to calm

Sixth Chakra: Ajna – Perception

Location: Between, in the center, and slightly above the line of the eyebrows.
Color: Indigo, Deep purple, or Dark plum. The skin vibrates purple.
Element: Beyond gross elements
Sense: Intuition
Qualities: Insight, Soul attached here, Where the inner teacher sits, Beyond duality, Oneness, Spirit,
Physical: Autonomic nervous system, Higher glands, Eyes, Brain
Unbalanced: Confusion, Unclear, Depression, Feeling "out of it," Lack of focus, Judgement
Balanced: Clear perception and vision, Reliable intuition, Focused, Complete, Comfort with self, Intuition is the voice of spirit, Inner-knowing
Yoga Postures: Forehead to the floor, Meditation
Foods: Purple grapes, Blackberries, Plums
Gemstones: Amethyst, Labradorite, Lapis Lazuli
Aromatherapy: Violet and Rose Geranium to stimulate, Hyacinth to calm

Seventh Chakra: Sahasrara – Infinite

Location: Crown of the head
Color: White or bright violet

Sense: Divine

Qualities: Container for life force, Recognition that we are one, Humility, Knowing, Vastness, Divine wisdom

Unbalanced: Doubt, Confusion, Denial of the spiritual realm, Religious extremism, Alienation, Fear of death, Ungrateful, Boastful

Balanced: Unity, Elevation, Bliss, Surrender, Connection, Conscious of the Infinite, Ability to let go, Empowered

Yoga Postures: Focus at the tip of the nose, Meditation

Gemstones: Selenite, Rainbow Moonstone, Clear Quartz

Aromatherapy: Violet and Amber to stimulate, Rosemary and Bergamot to calm

Additional: Sunshine, fresh air, and being out in nature is good for this chakra.

Eighth Chakra: Radiance

Location: Electromagnetic field, Aura, Weaves through the universe

Color: Projected from the chakras

Sense: Being

Qualities: Protects and projects, Positive attraction, Repels negativity, Buffer

Balanced: Filters out negative influences, Protection

Unbalanced: Withdrawn, Feeling vulnerable

Yoga Postures: Down-dog, Arm work, Meditation

Additional: To maintain vitality and range of color frequencies you need to stretch yourself by doing something new. Individual frequency needs to be higher than everything that moves through it. If you're not growing you lose aura and life force.

Chakras are independent but interconnected. It is my opinion that the combined unbalanced qualities listed for each chakra, gives a fairly accurate description of what it feels like to be stuck in active addiction. As we apply the principles of recovery and yoga the energy centers begin to balance and align to support better overall health.

The rainbow represents chakras one through seven, but each chakra also has its own rainbow of colors and any color may be found in any chakra. So, don't panic, there's nothing wrong if you are seeing colors in the chakras outside of the traditional rainbow representation. For instance, it is common for the fourth chakra to offer a glimpse of amber or pink, in addition to traditional green. Although I am presenting chakra commonalities, what we perceive in each energy center is as individual as each being.

The chakras can be seen as plug-in stations to the Universe, as the energy is not only contained within the body, but permeates the atmosphere around the body and beyond.

The circular spin of each chakra mimics the power pattern contained in the Buddhist rooted *Mandala*, which represents the whole circle of existence.

For the majority of the population, the chakras spin in a predictable direction when balanced. Exceptions to this basic rule do occur, but most follow the same rotation when they are in balance. If you are standing in front of your best friend, looking directly at the front of their body, the balanced chakra moves in a clockwise direction. Picture the hands of a clock circling around the belly button as if it is the center of the clock. Now you've located the third chakra. Balanced chakras all move in this direction; they don't switch their rotation as energy flows up the spine. Instead, they work as import and export stations, taking in and sending out energy like the flow of a river. Sometimes the river may move in a slow, lazy trickle, and other times it may roar and rush like it is being fed by fast melting snow. The strength and intensity of the river will change from day to day, season to season. As taught by healer Reverend Rosalyn Bruyere, energy flows through the chakras as concept, feeling, opinion, second feeling, response, insight, and release as we relate to both our inner and outer world.

Each of the five grossest elements also influence the chakras in the body, which in turn affect our thoughts, mood, and actions. There are many layers of elements; earth, water, fire, air, and ether form the substance for our experience. By substance I refer to what we would call matter, or what can be measured. The ether element, which relates to the higher chakras, actually penetrates all, so when we work on any of the four denser elements ether is also affected. Each element may be targeted based on current needs, to help build balance where desired in the chakra system. Simple suggestions may be taken to help balance each element as listed below.

Earth

Insecurity vs. Character and Faith
To balance the earth element, go out and literally connect with the earth. Walking barefoot on the earth, including dirt, grass, sand, forest, or desert will help to support a sense of being grounded and boost creativity.

Water

Lust vs. Integrity
To balance the water element, you'll want to submerge yourself in water. Take a dip in a lake, stream, pool, ocean, or even soak in a bathtub. Adding Epsom salt to your bath is especially helpful for cleansing and clearing the energy of the body.

<u>Fire</u>

Anger vs. Acceptance
This may sound paradoxical, but the sun helps to balance the fire element. Spend 20 minutes a day in the sun to boost immunity and balance the chakras. You can even go out in increments that add up to roughly 20 minutes. Make sure to break up the time if needed to avoid sunburn.

<u>Air</u>

Attachment vs. Happiness and Health
Pranayam, or breath work, helps to balance the air element in the body. There are many intentional *pranayam* exercises found within this book. Let's try one now.

Cycle of 4 breaths per minute

By consciously slowing down the rate of breath, positive changes happen in the body and mind. For example, by slowing the breath rate down to eight cycles per minute, healing, stress relief, relaxation, and mental awareness are all increased. Slowing the breath down to four cycles per minute adds increased mental function and sensitivity to the list of benefits already given. This four breath per minute cycle can be performed fairly easy by inhaling for five seconds, suspending the breath for five seconds, and exhaling for five seconds. Each breath should be complete and not rushed, moving between the nose and the navel. More detailed instruction is given on full yogic breathing in Chapter 4.

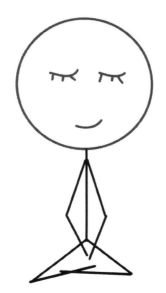

Mudras and Corresponding Chakras

Each of the fingers have pressure points that correspond to the chakras, in addition to our emotions, and the organs of the body. Hand positions that utilize pressure points at the tips of the fingers, or specific hand postures with connecting points, are called *mudras*. *Mudras* are commonly practiced in yoga and meditation. Pressure points that run along the length of the fingers are not as commonly used in yoga sets, but may be activated by holding the individual fingers one at a time. This can be done by wrapping the fingers of one hand around a single finger on the opposite hand. A simple meditation may be done on each of the fingers, using either the *mudra* or by activating the entire finger, while breathing long and deep. The pressure should be firm and cozy, but not cut off circulation. Hold for 1 to 3 minutes with an intentional long, deep breath.

Thumb – The thumb represents the earth and the ego and is associated with the 1st chakra. It provides a home base for the rest of the fingers to connect with for basic hand mudras.

Holding the thumb of each hand works on earth, ego, and the stomach. The pressure points stimulated along the thumb increase happiness and decrease worry.

Pointer – The index finger is the Jupiter finger and corresponds to the 4th chakra or heart center. Jupiter represents wisdom, knowledge, and expansion. It is also stormy and fun. Pressing the tip of the pointer finger to the tip of the thumb is called *Gyan Mudra* and basically translates as the hand position of wisdom.

Holding the pointer, or index finger, stimulates the kidneys and energetic expansion. The pressure points help to support knowledge and wisdom, and decrease fear.

Middle – The middle finger is the Saturn finger and it is influenced by the 3rd chakra. Saturn provides for an opportunity to practice patience, even in the presence of obstacles. It is a bit ironic that in our society people often use the middle finger when they are feeling most impatient. Pressing the tip of the middle finger to the tip of the thumb is called *Shuni Mudra*.

Holding the middle finger works on the liver, gallbladder, and inner fire of the 3rd chakra. Putting the squeeze on the middle finger increases patience, and decreases anger, shame, and frustration.

Ring – The ring finger is the Sun finger and it corresponds to the 2nd chakra which denotes flow. The Sun provides a warm, steady, vibrant energy that is anchoring. The energy is masculine in nature. Pressing the tip of the ring finger to the tip of the thumb is called *Surya Mudra*.

Holding the ring finger stimulates the lungs and large intestine. The pressure points activated along the finger promote a powerful, constant energy, and help to decrease sadness and depression.

Pinky – The pinky finger is the Mercury finger, and its super power is communication. The 5th chakra also represents communication. Pressing the tip of the pinky finger to the tip of the thumb is called *Buddhi Mudra.*

Holding the little finger corresponds to the pressure points of the heart and the small intestine. Activating these points increases intuition, communication, and healing, and decreases blame and judgement.

Palm of the hand – Holding the palm of the hand works on the 6th chakra for revitalization.

Illustrations of basic hand mudras

In getting to know your chakras, please don't feel like you have to digest this entire chapter at once; rather, experiment with the *mudras*, pressure points, elements, or breath meditation a little bit at a time. The intent of this chapter is to deliver a basic working knowledge of the chakras and easy practices to foster balance, in which the individual may choose to incorporate what is found to be helpful. Approach your exploration of the chakras with something that sparks your interest and try it on for size.

The Chakras

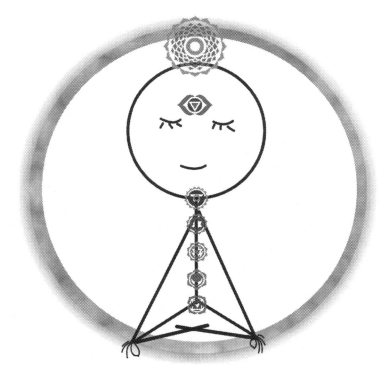

3

Eight Limbs of Yoga

What is Yoga?

Do I have to be able to contort myself in a pretzel to practice the poses? And, how in the world is putting my body into funny poses going to help me rediscover my spirit? Familiar questions? Read on to find out what's underneath the surface.

Yoga itself comes from the word *yoke*, which in the Hindu tradition implies union through physical and spiritual practice. By doing yoga, one helps to unite body, mind and spirit. From there, union can be extended to include the Divine. Time to throw in a disclaimer: yoga is a spiritual, not religious practice. It may help to think of it this way - religion takes place in a building, while spirituality is something God-given by virtue of being human. A yoga practice should support and enhance whatever your current beliefs and faith may be, and all denominations are welcome. There is no particular belief or faith required to practice yoga.

The history of yoga is much broader than a single person. Yoga is an ancient practice, dating back thousands of years, originally passed from teacher to disciple, maintaining an air of secrecy. The written record of yoga dates back approximately 2,000 years ago, when sage and yogi Maharishi Patanjali organized the yoga *sutras* to be passed on and preserved. The *sutras* are like packets of information detailing the lifestyle, practices, and benefits of yoga. The limbs given in this book come from the yoga *sutras*. The *sutras* are the first comprehensive written compilation of the complete yoga experience, detailing the prescribed practice for connecting to inner wisdom. Over the past 500 years, yoga has slowly made its way out of isolated pockets of humanity and into the service of humankind. During the last century yoga has evolved, coming into this age, spreading to benefit people worldwide.

Honestly, when I attended my first Kundalini yoga class, I felt like the teacher was speaking directly to me. The class had nothing to do with recovery or the 12 Steps, but the yoga principles blended seamlessly with the spiritual application of the steps, and over the months to follow yoga took my spiritual development to the next level. I personally continue to find yoga and meditation to be an amazing part of my ongoing recovery and growth. Bear with me through these next few chapters describing the foundation of yoga, as I intend to paint a picture that blends the spiritual principles of yoga and recovery.

The components of yoga are included in the eight limbs found within the yoga *sutras*. The limbs form the umbrella, and the branches fall under the umbrella embodying the different paths, or styles, of yoga.

The Branches and Limbs of Yoga

Branches:

As many as twenty-two styles of yoga fall under these six branches. I am including this list and a very brief description of each path solely for the purpose of providing a broad view of the scope of yoga. This book is based in the practice of Kundalini yoga. Kundalini yoga is considered primarily a Raj yoga, but within the practice can be found aspects of the other five branches. There are no harsh lines drawn between the paths, thus promoting an overlapping sense of unity.

Raja – Raj yoga is referred to as the royal path. The focus is on meditation. Traditionally this path called for a concentrated, monastic type of life, but we find its roots deeply imbedded in Kundalini yoga for modern times.

Bhakti – Bhakti is the path of devotion, commitment and total surrender to the love of the Divine. All is seen and done in service to the Divine.

Karma – Karma yoga is not about identifying the positive or negative actions we have taken, but rather identifying lessons from these actions which originate from a place of love. On the level of action, it is the path of service with the idea that what you do today creates your tomorrow. It is about giving selflessly without attachment.

Hatha – The focus is on the physical body. Posture and movement of the body are practiced to affect the mind and consciousness. Hatha yoga is based in posture, or *asana*.

Jnana – The building of knowledge inside oneself. This path is the path of intellectual study and analysis, including but not limited to, scripture.

Tantra – The yoga of ritual, and adopting beneficial rituals into daily life. Tantra is an easily misunderstood aspect of yoga because many associate it only with sex.

Eight Limbs of Yoga:

The eight limbs are equally essential in the process of discerning the real from the illusionary. They grow in relation to each other through the practice of yoga. Each limb is influenced by one of the three functional minds; negative, positive and neutral, and one of the five gross elements; earth, water, fire, air and ether.

1. Yama – Five Restraints
2. Niyama – Five Disciplines
3. Asana – Posture
4. Pranayama – Breath Work
5. Pratyhar – Synchronization
6. Dharana – Concentration
7. Dhyana – Meditation
8. Samadhi – Absorption in Spirit

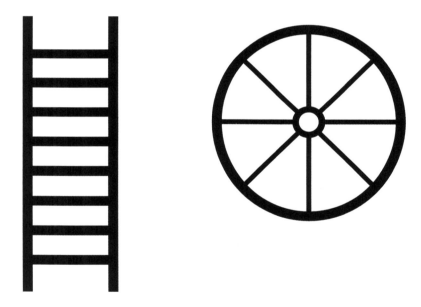

The eight limbs are described as eight spokes to the wheel. All of the spokes are needed for the complete experience, just as all the spokes of a wheel are needed to provide a smooth ride. Although all the spokes of the wheel are of equal importance, yoga typically has a starting point. It has been my experience that practitioners don't typically begin in absorption of spirit, but work toward a greater connection with spirit. It is with this frame of thought that I additionally like to visualize the eight limbs as a ladder. We begin at the bottom rung with our behavior and attitude and work our way up through posture, breath and meditation. First and foremost, we have to lay the foundation in our own outlook and action, and then can we begin to climb the ladder of growth and elevation to reach deeper states of meditation.

Yama – Five restraints

The *yamas* are influenced by the element earth. They outline the actions and attitudes to avoid in a way that grounds the individual, and challenges habits. I visualize *yama* as the stop sign, or as the red light at a traffic signal. The *yamas* tell us the behaviors to be avoided, but they are not written in the negative, they don't blatantly command don't do this or that. They offer an invitation for restraint, rather than a prohibition. The wording is given in terms of defining the desired moral behavior with an emphasis on competency. The *yamas* ask us to reflect on our true nature, our Divine nature.

Niyama – Five disciplines

The *niyamas* are influenced by water. They can be seen as the green light on the traffic signal, implying go. They encourage forward movement while implementing proper impulse control. Again, there is no direct order to conduct the self in alignment with these behaviors or attitudes, but rather a gentle recommendation. They are suggestions for behavior that imply personal responsibility and growth. The suggested disciplines are framed as a positive request. The *niyamas* ask us to evolve toward a harmony in all interactions, with the focus on duties and habits.

Asana – Postures for health and meditation

Asana is the limb of yoga that most people identify as "yoga." It is the actual physical posturing of the body. It is what you see pictured on the cover of fitness magazines or on TV. It is no doubt an essential part of yoga, but it is just one part of the whole. The element that influences *asana* is fire, supporting energy and action.

A deeper peek into *asana* shows that it allows the practitioner to prepare for meditation. In Kundalini yoga this is exactly what the exercise portion of class provides, a steady and relaxed body to sit more comfortably in meditation, with less distraction from the mind. *Asana* builds alertness and stability in the body and mind, and encourages an overall cohesion throughout all of the body's systems.

On a physiological level *asana* stimulates and purifies the systems in the body through its direct effect on the glands and organs, as well as muscle. An added bonus is that the physical movement and exertion helps to clear out intense, or even stagnant, emotions. *Asana* gives a physical outlet to cleanse body and mind.

Pranayam – Control of prana (life force), or "breath work"

Pranayam, or *pranayama* as it is called in some yoga traditions, is basically energy management. Through control of the breath, energy is directed throughout the body with intention. In yoga, one is asked to be mindful of every breath, not taking one single breath for granted. There are many different ways to perform yogic "breath work," but all of this work is within the realm of flow, suspension of the inhale or the exhale, release of the inhale or the exhale, and intention. *Pranayam* is influenced by the element of air, which gives expanded sensitivity within the breath.

Prana itself is Universal life force. *Prana* is not the breath, but the use of the breath does stimulate and circulate *prana* throughout the body. The circulation of *prana* through the body stimulates the body's systems, such as circulatory, endocrine, digestive, etc. *Prana* maintains the daily function of the body.

The following four limbs are influenced by the element of ether and exemplify sacred creative expression.

Pratyhar – Withdrawal of the senses

Pratyhar is synchronization with the senses as they draw inward. It is the practice of paying attention to sensory impulses in order to command the senses. Attention is intentionally focused on the sensory impulses by withdrawing from the outside. This inward focus allows one to hear the inner guiding voice with greater clarity. With practice the senses become disciplined so that they do not stray when the practitioner is consciously focusing.

The mind is easily distracted and will usually follow outside stimulation automatically; however, in *pratyhar* the mind holds steady. For instance, if the eyes see something bright and shiny, they will naturally wander on their own accord to investigate. They're like, "*Oh look, something shiny, let's check it out.*" It's an automatic sense response. In this example, while in the state of *pratyhar* the eyes will not wander off, but remain internally focused and synchronized with the mind, even when tempted by something bright and shiny. All of the other senses also behave in this way in the practice of this limb of yoga. They remain consolidated, dare I say well-behaved, within the individual practitioner.

Pratyhar is also an acknowledgment that all comes from the Divine. When one is in the state of *pratyhar* the Divine is acknowledged as the giver of all, and thanks are given with devotion. For a modern-day application, I like to use a sink full of dirty dishes to demonstrate the expression of *pratyhar*. I live with my husband and adult son and it seems like there are always dishes in the sink. Walking into a messy kitchen my first thought is usually something like, *"Evidently, I am the ONLY one in the house who knows how to do dishes.!"* Now, if I walk into the messy kitchen in a state of *pratyhar* my thought process would immediately be something along the lines of, *"How blessed we are to have dirty dishes in our sink, as God has given us plentiful food to place upon these dishes, running water to wash them, and a home to store the plates, so let us give thanks."* Can you see the difference?

A simple way to begin the process of going within is to spend some time just observing the mind each day.

Dharana – One-pointed concentration

Meditation focused on concentration, contemplation, attention, and intention describes the practice of *dharana*. It is a consistent penetration of thought and projectivity with consciousness. Meditating in this way supports change and healing. An actual practice can be holding the mind consciously on an object. For example, meditation done by focusing on an object, such as a flame or flower is a form of *dharana*. Below is a form of fixed gaze meditation called *Tratakum* that embraces *dharana*.

Tratakum meditation on a flame:

Sit in a comfortable seated posture with a straight spine, and place a candle on a table, or elevated surface, about 6 to 7 feet in front of your seated position. The flame should be at the level of the bridge of the nose. Gaze at the flame, focusing on the dark root of the fire for 3 to 11 minutes. Stay present as you focus on the flame. When the mind wanders or begins to tell you stories, gently bring the attention back to the flame. To end, inhale, exhale, and close the eyes, focusing at the brow for 1 minute.

Dhyana – Deep meditation

Dhyana is merger through meditation. The meditator is aware of witnessing thoughts but not involved. *Dhyana* is observation without attachment, which increases inner awareness and peace, and a broader sense of life. All things come and all things go.

"The only constant in life is perpetual change." -Deepak Chopra (2004)

A main difference between *dharana* and *dhyana* is the length of time spent in awareness. In *dharana* awareness moves in and out; it vacillates. In *dhyana* awareness remains steady for longer periods of time, and concentration is unbroken. In this relaxed state, pesky little things like stress, anxiety, irritation, or the screaming monkey mind are reduced. When in the deep state of dhyana, focus feels effortless.

Samadhi – Absorption in spirit

The highest state of meditation, or *samadhi*, can be seen as spiritual awakening. This is a state beyond time, of pure and unbounded awareness. This is who you really are, a knowing that you are a spiritual being having a human experience, not a human being having a spiritual experience. Words are hard to apply to *samadhi*, as it is an experience of direct knowledge and truth. This experience defies description.

It is my thought that as humans we may have glimpses of this true nature, brief experiences in this state, but we do not walk around functioning from this level in our daily unconscious living. States of *samadhi* may help in identifying the purpose of life. (I'll share a little secret here. In the teachings of Kundalini Yoga, it is said that the purpose of life is to enjoy it!)

"One of the deep truths captured by the eight limbs is the need to develop the entire spectrum of body and mind as a whole system. Kundalini Yoga includes all of the 8 limbs in each exercise set." -Gurucharan Singh Khalsa PhD (2003)

Yamas & Niyamas

The *yamas* and *niyamas* are defined as the five restraints and five disciplines. They outline a set of guidelines to live by. Below they are described in more detail, along with questions that are thought-provoking, and provide self-reflection as a guide for application in the modern world. It's time to get comfortable with the idea of self-evaluation. The reflection questions given below assist in the essential self-assessment found within the steps of recovery.

Yamas – The Five Restraints

Ahimsa

Ahimsa is translated as non-harming or non-hurting, but beyond that it is a development of loving kindness. It is fostering compassion, patience, love for self and others, and an understanding that all is one. This compassion is to encompass attitude and behavior. *Ahimsa* calls for a natural, delicate balance, and the ability to listen to the wisdom of the heart. In the book *How to Know God,* Sri Ramakrishna is quoted as explaining that true spirituality consists of *"making the heart and the lips the same."*

Ahimsa self-reflection:

Have I hurt another's feelings?
Is my self-talk supportive or defeating?

Do I gossip? (A side note about gossip; in the yogic teachings, it is said that when we gossip about another being, we take on their karma. Sometimes that thought alone reminds me to keep my mouth shut.)
Do I walk like I talk?
Am I living from a place of peace?
Do I recognize my participation in humanity as a whole?

Satya

Satya is translated as truthfulness. It is an ability to practice honesty, forgiveness, non-judgement, loving communication, and an integrity of thought, word, and action. Quite literally we are asked to speak the truth, and this includes owning our feelings. Logic resonates within *satya*, and we are challenged to distinguish between the observance (what we actually see), and the interpretation (how we respond, react, and relate to what we see). In all interactions there is a truth for the individuals involved, which may vary greatly because we all interpret and color events based on our current emotional state, and then there is the truth. The essence of truth comes from the heart and is embodied in the mantra *Sat Nam*. *Sat Nam* is translated as 'truth is my identity.'

<u>*Satya* self-reflection:</u>

I am trustworthy?
Do I ever tell white lies as a cover-up?
Do I know when to speak and when to be silent?
Do I make choices that are in line with my true, expanded self?
Do I hold grudges in the name of defending my interpretation of the truth?

Asteya

On the surface *asteya* is defined as non-stealing, but the deeper meaning is one of generosity. We are encouraged to heed the right use of resources, cultivate self-sufficiency, non-jealousy, and completeness within the self. *Asteya* supports an honest life based on connection to spirit, knowing that any outside possessions will not provide security and happiness. It invites us to radiate gratitude to support abundance. Rather than seeing ourselves as the owner of our "stuff" we can adopt the attitude of being the caretaker, as all things come and go. When we radiate generosity, prosperity is magnified.

This *yama* reminds me of a little story about free dessert. Are you the type of person who will accept a free dessert, even if you're not hungry and don't really desire it, just because it's free? Maybe you know someone like this? Many years back, I sat in a restaurant with a large group for dinner where one person in the group knew the restaurant manager. Due to this relationship, we were all offered free dessert at the end of our meal. Some were excited and grateful, some did not want dessert at all, and one person insisted the entire group should order dessert just because it was free. *"Take it, it's free!"* To this person there was no concern of desire or need; only the fact that it was free meant it should be taken. This story may be applied to any type of available offering, and is a reminder to take or use only what we need.

The nature of addiction is based in self-centeredness, greed, and in many ways getting needs met despite the effect on others. Reflecting often on the principle of *Asteya* ties naturally into the recovery process.

Asteya self-reflection:

Are there ways I can expand my generosity?
Am I pretending to be someone other than my authentic self?
Have I let go of fears relating to scarcity, loss, or not having enough?
Do I manipulate others to get my needs met?
Do I arrive on time and honor time boundaries?
Do I take more than I need?
Do I practice regular gratitude?

Bramacharya

On a primal level *bramacharya* is control of the senses, to include action taken, or action withheld, on said senses. It is sometimes translated as celibacy, but does not only apply to sexual activity. It is more accurately demonstrated through moderation and a healthy channeling of emotions. Attachments and dependency may be a challenge to finding the path of moderation and balance. *Bramacharya* asks us to align with our creative energy in a positive way, and to live our daily life as if it is sacred. Life is sacred. We strive for stability and balance while increasing life force, living with respect for body and mind, and expressing feelings appropriately.

The idea of moderating pleasure found through the senses may be a completely foreign concept to the practicing addict, and may feel counter-intuitive. This will change with growth in recovery, but may never feel easy. That's ok. Start slowly by picking one thing from the list below to approach with greater awareness and mindfulness.

Bramacharya self-reflection:

Do I moderate all sense pleasures?
Do I moderate the use of my energy?

Does my energy swing between high and low extremes of all or nothing?

Can I find pleasure in the simplicity of spirit?

Do I require more moderation in food, work, TV, relationships, etc.?

Am I able to self-correct my behavior?

Do I offer honor and respect in my interactions with others?

Aparigraha

Aparigraha is defined as non-possessiveness. At its center, it is acknowledging abundance in life's ebb and flow with a deep sense of gratitude. Personal awareness is expanded to include less attachment and possessiveness to the material world. In the absence of aversion and attachment, jealousy lessens and peace is found in the essential nature of the self. One fulfills needs rather than wants, and is able to distinguish the difference between them. *Aparigraha* is not really about possessions, but rather the attitude toward them. It fosters the development of relationships with self and others that include healthy boundaries. When we give to others out of generosity it should be a token of genuine affection, not because we expect something in return. Cultivate an attitude of *"I am enough,"* and find the blessing in all.

When one personally connects with the concept of *"I am enough,"* the impulse to take things and/or people hostage in order to quell internal insecurities lessens. The need to find outside approval for validation decreases as self-fulfillment is experienced.

Aparigraha self-reflection:

Am I willing to let go?

Am I judgmental?

Do I trade my inner peace or my health for material things?

Do I take advantage of others, or have I cultivated the practice of self-reliance?

Am I grateful for my home, food, and surroundings?

Am I being of service?

Do I know the difference between my wants and my needs?

Niyamas – The Five Disciplines

Shaucha

Shaucha is translated as purity, an evenness of mind, thought and speech. In addition, it is purity of body both in terms of nourishment and physical and mental cleanliness. Toxic intake is to be avoided. In *shaucha* we strive to overcome negative or hurtful thoughts as well as actions, and cultivate the joyful nature of being human. Positive affirmations can be a simple action step toward redirecting negative thoughts. It is beneficial to be part of a spiritual community or fellowship of like-minded people. A longing for simplicity and purity of heart are developed through the practice of *shaucha*.

This is an opportunity to honestly evaluate personal self-care. The list below may feel extreme in suggesting clean body, mind, food, and self-talk, but feel free to take baby steps. Begin with one reflection on the list.

Shaucha self-reflection:

Am I physically clean and neat?
Do I eat clean food?
Do I purify emotions?
Do I indulge in negative self-talk?
Do I entertain negative thoughts about others?
Have I built a spiritually supportive community?
Do I keep it simple?

Santosha

Santosha means contentment. It is a cultivating of gratitude, acceptance, and calmness in the face of success or failure. *Santosha* is an invitation to be aware in the present moment, welcome all experiences as part of life, and an acceptance of what is. It is a peace that is absent of addiction and is not dependent on surrounding circumstances. As faith grows, satisfaction comes from within, affording an acceptance of life on life's terms, and enabling a release of regrets from the past and a letting go of worry over the future. We develop a sense of duty to help others. *Santosha* is a state of deep satisfaction and appreciation regardless of external circumstances. Overall, *santosha* is about being deeply content from the inside out.

Santosha self-reflection:

Do I live with passion?
Do I have gratitude?
Do I feel content?
Do I release expectations in order to experience freedom?
Am I dependent upon other people, places, or things for personal peace?
Does my behavior support all living beings on the planet?
Am I able to accept life on life's terms?

Tapas

Tapas is about purification and living life with zeal, or great energy, courage, and enthusiasm. It is the power of refinement through determination and willingness for practices. What kind of practices? Well since this *Niyama* is included in the eight limbs of yoga, *tapas* in motion refers to the repetition of meditation, and embracing transformation through action. The repetitive action of meditation helps to create harmony, virtue, and reverence in our attitude toward all. The fire and passion found in *tapas* supports consistency and perseverance in building healthy habits.

Interestingly, many people new into recovery think that as they "clean up" or "purify" their lives, they will be bored and boring. It's almost as if purification and living life with zeal and passionate enthusiasm are believed to be mutually exclusive. Well, I'm here to tell you they are not. When we burn off the debris, we are free to live our best life, chase our dreams, and help others, all while maintaining discipline.

Tapas self-reflection:

Do I keep commitments?
Do I practice self-discipline; physical, mental and emotional?
Do I have a regular meditation practice?
Do I pay attention to my words?
Do I feel passionate about my goals?

Svadhyaya

Svadhyaya is defined as study, and in a deeper sense utilizing reflection and meditation to expand knowledge. *Svadhyaya* is not only about reading and studying writings of a spiritual nature, but also a looking within, self-study, and introspection. Self-study is to be conducted without judgement. Discernment is used when observing, listening, and seeking information. Self-value comes from within, from connection to spirit, rather than outside influences.

The gathering of information has changed radically over the past century. In our modern world you can read more information in one day than the average person would read during their entire lifetime just 100 years ago. Wow! In the past people have been ridiculed, punished, and even burned at the stake for discoveries we now take for granted as the truth. The process of communicating information is ever evolving. Today we have the entire web available at our fingertips. We can literally call up almost anything we want to know in a matter of seconds. *Svadhyaya* asks us to use discernment and wisdom in this big, wide world of information.

Svadhyaya self-reflection:

Do I confuse information with wisdom?
Do I use my yoga and meditation practice for insight into how to live daily life?
Do I learn from past mistakes?
Do I practice regular journaling?
Am I taking regular personal inventory?

Ishvara Pranidhana

Ishvara Pranidhana is whole hearted dedication, devotion, and surrender to the Divine. It's a matter of living in the moment with faith and dedication, free from attachments. *Ishvara Pranidhana* is a devotion so strong that as awareness of the personal journey increases, peace can be found even in uncertainty. It calls forth the heart center for wisdom, clarity, and trust. A personal relationship with prayer may be expressed in alignment with each individual's beliefs and experiences. Humility is a natural by-product when the ego is surrendered to Source and the feet are firmly grounded in the search for truth.

The principles of *ishvara pranidhana* echo through steps 3, 7, 11 and 12, which rely on surrender and connection to something greater than the self as a solution to the malady of addiction.

Ishvara Pranidhana self-reflection:

Am I willing to allow daily activities to flow from love?
Do I ask for help only when desperate, or am I open to support and growth?
Do I accept the consequences of my behavior?
Am I able to take action and let go of the results?
Do I have a personal prayer?

Take a few moments to write a personal affirmation:

The 8 Limbs of Yoga

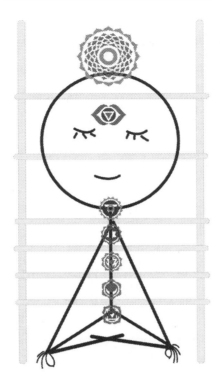

4

Ten Energy Bodies

Did you know we actually have more than one body? We have a total of ten! The ten light, or energy, bodies are located in and around the physical body. The physical body is one of our ten bodies, and provides the vehicle for the other nine energy bodies to play out their parts. We process all information and experience, the full spectrum of life, through the ten bodies.

"Many philosophical traditions divide the whole person into three aspects: body, mind, and spirit. The ten bodies are a refinement of this breakdown. The physical body is single in both traditions. But, instead of one "mind," there are three, each with a different aspect of how the mind works (negative, positive, and neutral). Instead of "spirit" being a blanket description of all of the subtle or energetic parts of our being, in the ten body system there are six different aspects of our "spirit," each with a significantly different purpose (arcline, aura, soul, pranic, subtle, and radiant). Having ten ways of looking at our experience instead of three gives a richer understanding of who we are and how we relate to the world around us." - Santokh S. Khalsa DC (2021)

Soul Body

The soul is the first of the ten bodies, and it is a word with a familiar connotation. Many traditions believe in the soul. The soul body is humble, heart-centered, and creative. The soul is a spark in the heart center, an inner guiding light, and can be your best friend. The soul allows for the individual expression of the spirit that resides within each of us. This is the energy body that longs for connection, communion with the Divine, and drives personal desire to search and grow.

The soul body responds to work on the first chakra because its challenge and weakness may be feeling stuck, lacking purpose, and coming from the head rather than the heart. The identified challenge is true for the disease of addiction as well, and it is imperative to move beyond the head and into the heart. It is important to define what aspect of the self is running the show, who is in charge, the soul or the ego. Should the answer be the ego, difficulty and struggle are sure to follow. In the yogic teachings, it is clear that for a happy life the soul is to be in charge, not the mind or ego. They are the servants. To inspire the soul body, raise the Kundalini energy consciously through yoga.

The soul body has great sensitivity and penetration, living throughout all of the five elements: ether, air, fire, water, and earth. The following nine energetic bodies were given to serve the soul.

Negative Mind

The negative mind is the second energy body, and the first of the mental bodies. The negative mind is the primal discerning mind, designed to detect danger and keep us safe. Its primary concern is survival. This mind is the first aspect to process incoming information for the purpose of protection and containment. It has a drive to connect with a Higher Power and guidance from within, but by nature is defensive, doubting and skeptical. This is the mind that will tell you to "STOP" before reacting. Even though its job is to survey and calculate, this built-in stop sign provides a positive pause for deeper evaluation.

The challenge for the negative mind is not to give in to a negative attitude or unhealthy or self-destructive relationships, and to overcome obstacles to trust. Don't let this mind talk you out of doing something that would be beneficial. Balance in the second chakra is helpful in supporting a healthy negative mind through self-discipline, building healthy relationships and community, and developing integrity.

Positive Mind

The positive mind is the third energy body, and the second of the mental bodies. The positive mind resonates with desire, and it is the mind that encourages us to follow our dreams and goals. It seeks potential, assesses benefits, and finds fulfillment as it processes incoming information. It is optimistic, playful, powerful yet humble, and explores all possibilities. This is the mind that will tell you to "GO." I think of this mind as our own personal cheerleader. This mind sees opportunity and predicts success.

I ran across a very interesting statement about the positive mind in *Senses of the Soul* by GuruMeher Khalsa (2013). He states, *"When it (the positive mind) takes over, desire is misused for protection, and you can get lost in fantasy and drown in excess. Without the balance of the protective (negative) mind, obsession and addiction feel 'safe' but create danger."*

Challenges faced by an under-developed positive mind are feelings of fear, being overwhelmed, depressed, and giving up. Stay in the present moment to avoid being sucked back into the past where this mind can draw information out of the subconscious mind and apply it to the now. To support the positive mind, work on the navel center, or third chakra, to improve self-esteem. This can be done physically by working the abdomen with yoga, and mentally by practicing positive affirmations.

Neutral Mind

The neutral mind is the fourth energy body, and the third aspect of the mind or mental body. The neutral mind is the conscious mind and the ultimate decision maker. It weighs the pros and cons of the negative and positive minds, sorts through information, and makes a decision based on our highest good and an effortless win-win outcome. It is comprehensive, provides guidance, and functions in relation to time and space. It also has the ability to see the bigger picture. The neutral mind is developed through meditation which cultivates compassionate intuition and guidance. It ultimately wants what is best for all, and may be referred to as the "wise judge."

The challenges facing the neutral mind are underdeveloped, or unbalanced, negative or positive minds. The neutral mind may have difficulty deciphering clear information and vacillate between the input of the negative and positive minds, struggling to make decisions. Playing the victim is also a weakness for this fourth energy body. The solution for strengthening the neutral mind is meditation.

Before moving on to the fifth body, I would like to make additional comments about the negative, positive, and neutral minds and their relationship. First of all, I'd like you to think of the mind as a full body phenomenon, not something that takes place only in the brain. The three functional minds, or mental bodies, permeate the entire being and influence the way we behave and interact with others.

The negative mind does not necessarily correspond to having a negative attitude; its purpose is to provide protection. If the negative mind is over-developed and projecting too strongly, it can prevent us from taking any action out of fear of harm or failure. When out of balance this mind may reflect the world as a scary place, and we may in fact demonstrate a negative attitude. If the negative mind is under-developed, we may lack the ability to ascertain danger and project a lackadaisical outlook on life. A balanced negative mind uses judgement to provide a proper evaluation of risk and supports appropriate action.

It is also true that the positive mind does not translate as having a positive attitude, but rather it provides an optimistic evaluation of potential gains in any given situation. If the positive mind is over-developed, the expression may simulate a positive attitude and the portrayal of being up for anything. This over-developed positive mind carries the risk of being blindsided by life's difficulties due to a lack of awareness that danger could even possibly exist, let alone be present on a personal level. An under-developed positive mind may undermine personal goals and dreams by discounting them, or it may present as a lack of energy and drive.

The neutral mind, also known as the meditative mind, resides in the heart center, which is a space of transition, calm, neutrality, and clarity. The neutral mind literally sifts through the pros and cons from both the negative and positive minds, and its job is to make a neutral decision based on the middle path. This middle road concept is also known as *Dharma*, which translates as the righteous path. Walking a dharmic path is designed to keep us on the neutral path to avoid swinging from one extreme to the other. If the neutral mind is over- or under-developed, it may be swayed, or even bossed around, by either the negative or positive mind. For our overall well-being, it is important that the neutral mind be balanced. To reiterate, this balance is attained through meditation.

Meditation may reveal what is needed for balance in each mind; for instance, do we need to find our voice and use it, or do we need to pause and be silent? There is no *"one size fits all"* journey.

As information is received and a decision is to be made, there is no side stepping any of the three functional minds. Although they each have their own characteristics and duties, they very much function as one team. Incoming information runs through the three minds in a loop, always in the order of negative, positive, and neutral, and it only takes 9 seconds to complete this loop. In my yoga classes I often suggest to students that when they find themselves immediately offended by people, places, or things, they simply close the mouth and let the 9 seconds run its course. In this way one can avoid reacting from the negative mind only. If the full process is allowed to run through, it is more probable that we may act consciously, rather than react in a knee-jerk fashion. This can keep us from having to make amends later down the line.

Yoga does not demand perfect execution in balancing the aspects of the mind. It shares knowledge and asks us to investigate and experiment for ourselves. You can view the functional minds as having your back if you do your part to take care of them through meditating and inner-listening. In a later chapter on the twelve steps, we'll take a look at how to do things differently when we find we are unable to think our way out of situations or problems that our own thinking got us into in the first place. Meditation can be applied as a solution in that it provides an interruption, or intervention, if you will, to our usual repetitive thought process. It helps to calm and consolidate the three minds, and offers us a heart-centered answer. The middle road may sound boring, but it's simply eliminating the drama as we step into the happy, fun, maybe slightly neurotic, free, authentic self.

Physical Body

The physical body is the fifth energy body. It is the body that people relate to, and usually the only one they think they have. This body houses the five senses - sight, sound, taste, touch, and smell, and it is where pain and pleasure are communicated. It is tangible. It moves, feels, interprets and shares our life experiences. The physical body is given as our personal temple to navigate this journey on earth. This body is our teacher, and it dominates our perception of life. Viewed as our own personal temple, yoga asks us to take care of the body physically, mentally, emotionally, and spiritually.

Ask yourself, "Am I taking better care of my car than myself?" Do you put gas in the tank when needed, keep the tires filled with air, perform regular maintenance and repairs, and keep it clean? Are you doing the same for your physical body, including getting proper rest and eating a healthy diet? The physical body craves balance. Troubles with the fifth body may correspond to the fifth chakra manifesting as difficulty expressing the self, anger, and feeling like life is a competition. To help correct discontent in the physical body it is important to find your inner teacher, and maybe even literally teach something - macrame, the steps, English 101, how to change a tire, anything that is of interest. Discipline, especially in the areas of exercise and meditation are also important for keeping the physical body aligned and functioning well. The true beauty of the human body radiates from within.

Arc Line

The arc line is the sixth energy body, an energetic ring that extends from one ear lobe, up over the head, to the other ear lobe. It is a dense expression of energy over the head that ties into the power of projection. The arc line intensifies the projection of ideas, thoughts, prayer, and meditation. It attunes to balance between the physical and cosmic realms, and increases concentration, focus, and intuition to help deal with external and internal life stressors. The arc line gauges the individual level of energy and provides calm and graceful guidance within the aura.

It is said that the *Akashic* record is stored in the arc line, within the aura. Over simplified, the *Akashic* record contains information about all of our lives, past and present actions, and all owed or accrued karma. The yogic teachings indicate that our destiny is written on the arc line. We are called to live our destiny or suffer our fate.

The arc line ties into the sixth chakra, or third eye, and has a direct relationship with the pituitary gland. The pituitary gland is the master gland in the body. Distant, silent messages may be received at this center, and this is not as far out as it may sound. These messages may seem like they come out of nowhere as a thought, a dream, or an inner knowing that you just have to take a particular action or say something specific to someone. This is subtle communication, or intuition, delivered through the sixth energetic body.

Awakening and balancing the sixth chakra and body is achieved through meditation, which in turn decreases mood swings and being overpowered by outside influences. Meditation also helps to develop strong intuition.

Auric Body

The aura is the seventh energy body. The aura or magnetic field interacts with the world and provides a buffer between the physical body and the surrounding environment. It is basically a container for life force, inner strength and vitality. Its job is to protect and filter energy coming into the individual field in the present moment.

As mentioned in Chapter 2, the use of chemicals and addictive behavior is damaging to the aura. Fortunately, yoga and meditation help to cleanse, strengthen and repair the aura.

The seventh chakra is also related to the aura. Meditation works to keep the aura strong, repelling dis-ease and negativity. Meditation also helps to overcome challenges to the aura, as well as the arc line, attracting positivity into the field. The strength of the aura is a reflection of the individual's inner health, as well as external behavior.

Pranic Body

The *pranic* body is the eighth energy body and it corresponds to the Infinite. *Prana* is translated as life force. This body gives life, and is our own inner healer. Breath penetrates every cell and acts as a conductor for *prana* to circulate throughout the body, thus stimulating all of its internal systems. The *pranic* body can be thought of as the spiritual warrior. It allows us to feel motivated, alive, and provides energy to achieve goals in life.

Pranayam, or breath work, is the solution to challenges for the *pranic* body such as feelings of fear, fatigue, defensiveness, or anxiety. The breath is the key to access healing in the body. The breath is the way in to the body, mind, and spirit. Deep breathing specifically will help to balance *prana*. It's time to circulate prana.

Long Deep/Yogic Breathing

A full yogic breath is helpful for creating calm and healing. This may be done in Easy Pose, or an alternative seated posture. Allow yourself to observe the breath coming in and out through the nose, without changing anything. Breathing through the nose is important because the air coming in is cleansed and hydrated through the nose.

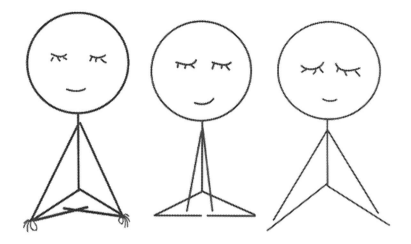

As you observe your breath, slowly bring your attention to your belly, and on the inhale bring the breath down to the navel and gently expand your belly. Release the breath, letting all of the air go. Make sure you exhale completely before taking a new, fresh and complete inhale. As you inhale again, slowly expand the belly, and bring the expansion up to fill the lower lobes of the lungs. Exhale completely. This time expand the breath even further, creating a three-part wave. Inhale, the wave begins to swell in your belly, draw it up expanding the lower lobes of the lungs, and bring it up throughout the lungs all the way up to the collarbone. Release the breath from the collarbone, down through the lungs, and lastly let the navel move gently toward the spine as all of the air is expelled. It may be helpful to think of taking a wide inhale and a tall exhale. Continue inhaling and exhaling in this three-part wave for 3 to 11 minutes. If you are new to full yogic breathing and you begin to feel light-headed or dizzy, ease up a bit. This may be a totally new approach to the breath and oxygenating the body. The breath should not be forced but allowed to flow.

Benefits of Long Deep Breathing/Yogic Breathing

- Increased oxygenation
- Impacts detoxification of the organs
- Improves function of the respiratory system
- Reduces cortisol and adrenaline

- Lowers blood pressure
- Lowers heart rate
- Helps to balance the nervous system
- Increases feelings of relaxation and calm in the body and mind
- Releases stress and tension
- Increases awareness and clarity
- Boosts energy
- Increases concentration
- Increases the flow of prana and overall circulation
- Promotes health and vitality
- Promotes positive support in mental function
- Improved sleep

Subtle Body

The subtle body is the ninth energy body. It is the most difficult to sense because it is fragile, transparent, and light. It is delicate and cues us into the subtleties and nuances of life. The etheric nature of the subtle body enables us to learn quickly, be calm, and intuitively know what is going on in any situation. It has an intertwined relationship with the soul and in yogic philosophy it is said to carry the soul through transition at the time of earthly passing. It is the most powerful guardian.

The challenge of the subtle body is to stay connected to true purpose in life, overcoming foolishness and immaturity to remain self-aware. To strengthen the subtle body, it is recommended to meditate for one thousand consecutive days.

Additionally, the subtle body may be supported by submersing yourself in beauty, either through your own creative flow or through visiting inspiring environments.

Also try decluttering your environment and getting rid of objects that are not joyful or useful. Clutter is an extension of personal energy, so it is beneficial to clean up spaces where time is spent, such as home, work, and car.

Radiant Body

The radiant body is the tenth and final energy body, and the highest manifestation of our human condition. It asks for us to give it our all and always be courageous. This body ties into our own inner radiance, or royalty, the light that shines through. If you have met someone you would describe as charismatic, it is the radiant body you are sensing. The radiant body is all about magnetic attraction. Yoga invites us to let our inner light shine big and bright, to use our energy to attract rather than pursue.

Our light shines not to cast shadows, but to uplift and lighten those around us for the benefit of all. This body emanates courage and confidence. Whereas the other nine bodies are receptive, the radiant body projects energy.

If you find yourself to be fearful, reserved, or lacking responsibility, it is recommended to make a commitment of some type. Following through with commitment builds the radiant body. This ties in beautifully to the 12 Step program where making commitments to others and the fellowship is a huge part of the recovery process and is actually a part of taking care of the self.

The 10 Bodies

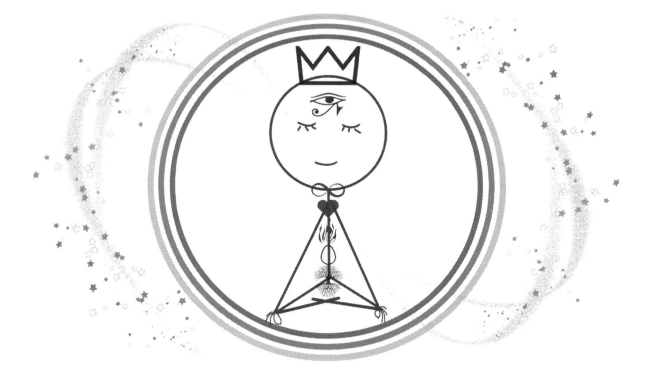

5

The Twelve Steps

I am choosing to present the Twelve Steps of Narcotics Anonymous because they are all inclusive, and although the identified word describing the addiction may vary from program to program, the steps are the same through all anonymous programs. There is no specific substance or behavior assigned within these steps. The identified problem is personal for each individual, and these steps simply refer to addiction.

The Twelve Steps of Narcotics Anonymous

1. We admitted that we were powerless over our addiction, that our lives had become unmanageable.
2. We came to believe that a Power Greater than ourselves could restore us to sanity.
3. We made a decision to turn our will and our lives over to the care of God as we understood Him.
4. We made a searching and fearless moral inventory of ourselves.
5. We admitted to God, to ourselves, and to another human being the exact nature of our wrongs.
6. We were entirely ready to have God remove all these defects of character.
7. We humbly asked Him to remove our shortcomings.
8. We made a list of all persons we had harmed, and became willing to make amends to them all.
9. We made direct amends to such people wherever possible, except when to do so would injure them or others.
10. We continued to take personal inventory and when we were wrong promptly admitted it.
11. We sought through prayer and meditation to improve our conscious contact with God as we understood Him, praying only for knowledge of His will for us and the power to carry that out.
12. Having had a spiritual awakening as a result of these steps, we tried to carry this message to addicts, and to practice these principles in all our affairs.

Principles of the 12 Steps

1. Honesty
2. Hope
3. Faith
4. Courage
5. Integrity
6. Willingness
7. Humility
8. Responsibility
9. Discipline
10. Perseverance
11. Awareness
12. Service

The various 12 Step programs available for self-help today have been adopted and adapted from the founding 12 Step program of Alcoholics Anonymous. The program suggests working the steps in order to achieve freedom from active addiction, the bondage of self, and to progress in personal growth and recovery. The steps are usually worked with a sponsor, for the purpose of support and guidance along the way. A sponsor is someone who has experience working the steps and has typically been clean, sober, and/or in recovery longer than the person they are assisting.

I used to think it was crazy that the solution to addiction is a set of steps written in a book. Really, if I read this list, it will change my life?! What I found is that it's not really about the reading. There's application, footwork, study, honest self-appraisal, making the conscious decision to do things differently, and a challenging of old beliefs. It is through action that the steps come alive. They come off of the pages and into life. This is the divine magic found within the twelve steps.

If you are in recovery yourself, absorb and apply what you can use. If you are a yoga teacher reading this, wanting to teach a class to a recovering population, my hope is that this gives you a better understanding of the disease concept in addition to the process your students in recovery will be walking through. Willingness to try new things and be open-minded may be affected by the length of time a student has been in recovery. Those newer to being clean and sober may show more resistance to a yoga practice; they're just learning the ropes and getting to know themselves so to speak, whereas those who are seasoned recovery veterans may take naturally to yoga and meditation. In treatment settings, I suggest a gentle approach. One of the best benefits yoga can offer individuals in any type of residential treatment center is relaxation.

If you are teaching in treatment centers, or addicts new to recovery, your students are looking for camaraderie and connection. Those who are brand new do not yet know this and may immediately deny it, believing themselves to be self-sufficient. Yoga teachers may come up against rigid thinking and what feels like a brick wall. I suggest showing up as your authentic self and presenting the yoga and meditation without an agenda to sell the practice; simply deliver the teachings. I have a few stories that stand out from my time teaching in a treatment center for male parolees coming out of the prison system, and I'll share one of them now.

One afternoon while teaching in the treatment center I could tell that the group was not into the practice, so I began talking to them while doing gentle stretches. They still had the walls up, so I got them on their feet for some forward folds. In the process of folding forward my t-shirt lifted a tiny bit, exposing a small portion of a tattoo I have on the front side. That was all it took for them to feel a connection, to feel that they were understood and accepted. One of the men pointed his finger at me and loudly declared, "*She has a tattoo.*" The room shifted immediately to warmth and openness, they were asking questions and participating. I'm certainly not suggesting you need to get a tattoo to connect with any particular group, but just know your target audience wants to feel accepted and understood. They may be starved for human comfort and not even know it. Whatever the population, from parolee to entitled brat, the answer is love and acceptance, and don't forget to bring your boundaries.

Whether you are applying this book for personal practice and growth, or interested in learning about the topic of yoga and recovery, or you're going to teach yoga to recovering people, rule number one is to go with the flow. Great plans are often derailed, and flexibility is needed as we continue on our path. Maintaining an open and flexible mind allows for an identification with similarities, rather than a search for differences. Both yoga and recovery seek communion.

As with chakras, *sutras*, and bodies there is a natural forward progression in the steps. There is a beautiful simplicity in the flow. Yes, simple, but not necessarily easy. It can be quite painful to take an honest look at the self. However, it is a path out of self-induced misery. The steps can be viewed like the ladder given in the earlier chapter on the eight limbs of yoga. Step work is progressive. A popular program slogan shared in days gone by states, "*The elevator to recovery is broken, take the steps.*" There are no free rides.

The twelve steps outline a self-applied, peer-supported program for recovery. The model is community-based and focuses on healing the whole being through active accountability and change of behavior.

The 12 Steps provide a spiritual solution to a problem that manifests outwardly physically, mentally, and emotionally. The freedom of choice inherent in the steps allows for an integration into any lifestyle. Although it is a spiritual program, there is no specific belief required to work the steps, just as no particular belief is required to practice yoga. The gift of the steps is a road to self-discovery and growth.

The road traveled in recovery delivers a deepened interaction with self and with a power greater than self, paralleling the journey through the eight limbs of yoga. Both the steps and the limbs imply building a relationship with the nature of God, or an absorption with spirit. We are not asked to jump right in to this relationship, but rather dip our toes in the water and try it out. We begin with working on our own thoughts and behavior before getting cozy with a power greater than ourselves. For those who struggle with the concept of God, I like to recommend to just get over the word. Let it go for now.

In any 12 Step program, God may represent willingness to be open to taking Good, Orderly Direction. It's about being open to something new and different than our old ways. For those who are in self-will run riot, this new perspective can be a saving grace. In yoga, God is described as the Generating, Organizing, and Destroying energies found in all beings. These principles exist inherently in all of us as the expression of the Divine.

The beauty of both is that you can choose your own personal relationship with the God of your understanding. Whether you ever choose to use the word God or not, the verbiage in the steps indicates a progression in the relationship with a Higher Power. The words themselves denote a personal, warm, developing relationship beginning with a Power Greater than the self, to a Higher Power, then to God, and lastly Him (or whatever gender pronoun you prefer).

If you are bristling, again, I'll ask you again to let go of the word "God," or "Him." In the English language when we use the third person plural pronoun "they", there is no gender, but the singular use has traditionally been masculine. Please feel free to substitute with Goddess, Her, They or any name or pronoun meaningful to you. No one defines your relationship with a Higher Power but you! For some people it comes from a religion or tradition they grew up with, for some it is nature, for others it is the logic of mathematics. No matter the concept of a Higher Power, a thorough working of the steps is an unveiling and discovery of the true inner nature of being human.

I have worked in and around chemical dependency treatment for over three decades, and I have yet to see an approach outside of the Twelve Step fellowships to be more successful for long-term recovery. It is in the spirit of recovery and freedom that I share the natural weave of energy and principles between the steps, chakras, yoga limbs, and energetic bodies in this book. When we get to the chapter on individual steps and the yoga sets recommended to support the step work, I will be sharing, as I am now, from both a recovery and yogic point of view.

The progression through the stages of recovery is listed as identified by Terrance T. Gorski and Merlene Miller in *Staying Sober (1986)*. The following six stages have no set time frame for each stage. Individuals move through this growth process at their own pace. I am sharing these stages to demonstrate the natural flow of growth, but I would like to note that these stages come from my days working as a chemical dependency counselor; they are not stated or written in the 12 Step programs. There is a fine line to be walked between treatment and the anonymous programs of recovery. They are completely autonomous, but complementary, and I am sharing a bit of both as we move through the steps because it is my personal background. Knowledge and awareness of the journey ahead can be helpful in walking the path.

The six stages of recovery:

1. Pretreatment
2. Stabilization
3. Early Recovery
4. Middle Recovery
5. Late Recovery
6. Maintenance

Pretreatment

1. Realization that something is not right through thought, emotion, or circumstance.
2. Transition into awareness that using substances creates negative consequences.
3. Questioning whether addiction could be the problem or abstinence could be the solution.
4. Rationalizing the questions away. *"Yeah but, … If only."*
5. Shock. May be forced into abstinence by family, friends, situations, or the law.

Stabilization

1. The processes of judgment, behavior, and emotions begin to stabilize.
2. Interrupt the pattern of addiction.

3. Recognize addiction and possible solutions.
4. Clarity of thought begins to return.

Early Recovery

1. Structure is essential for supporting the recovery process.
2. Admission and relation to symptoms of addiction.
3. Accept help, 12 Step programs, therapy, begin to share, and learn tools for recovery.
4. Movement from intellectual compliance of *I think I'm an addict*, to acceptance of addition and willingness to try the program.
5. The greater involvement and investment, the deeper the recovery.

Middle Recovery

1. Work on stability and balance in all areas of life.
2. Lifestyle shifts, drug-centered to recovery-centered.
3. Willingness to change increases.
4. Helping others and allowing others to help oneself.

Late Recovery

1. Discovery: Who am I? What do I like? What do I believe?
2. Continuous problem solving. The only thing you can count on is change.
3. Stress management. HALT, don't get too hungry, angry, lonely, or tired.
4. Deep healing of childhood issues, emotional development and maturity.
5. Freedom to live life.

Maintenance

1. Maintenance supports a meaningful life, not just survival.
2. Maintain an effective recovery program.
3. Live with a strong maintenance program to prevent relapse.

To reiterate, there is not a fixed time period given to any stage. Individuals move through the stages at their own pace. This happens organically; there's no checklist for addicts to mark the boxes that indicate moving to the next stage; it just happens. Rough times, or complacency, can occur in any stage and they can be a normal part of recovery. There are warning signs that action is required to get back on track, and they can manifest as boredom, replacing addiction of choice with other activity, depression, irritability, cockiness, loneliness, superficial interaction with others, or becoming withdrawn and isolated. These feelings and behaviors are messages, indicators that a change in direction is required. Recovery is action based.

I would like to return to the "*Yeah, but…*" rationale mentioned above in the pre-treatment stage of recovery. This mindset attempts to divert and deny personal accountability for current circumstances, and may carry over, or even return, into later stages of recovery. It is usually an expression of feeling different than others, or self-pity, and/or that life is not fair. "Yeah, but" creates a personal road block, and should be challenged.

Experiment shifting the thought process of "yeah, but" by saying or thinking "yes, and." This is actually a suggestion adapted from a theatre game by the same name. "Yeah, but" justifies a poor-me attitude, whereas "yes, and" invites elaboration, and a richness of exploration. Don't sell yourself short, a new life is worth taking the time to investigate and create.

The recovery process gives instruction to build a foundation by beginning to work on the internal aspects that fuel our addictions – our thoughts, attitudes, and behaviors. Then it moves on to deal with external relationships and wreckage created while under the influence. Lastly, the 12 Steps suggest maintaining spiritual fitness and self-accountability. Steps 1 through 3 ask the addict to honestly look at the self, make a commitment, and then dive deep into healing. Steps 4 through 9 ask the addict to do the work involved in personal healing. This includes the internal self-care needed to stay clean, and then the action to amend relationships and outward behavior. Steps 10 through 12 are the maintenance steps, which allow for continuous review of personal recovery. The foundation is laid brick by brick. It is a process, not something that happens all at once. The yogic ladder given in Chapter 3 reflects the idea of building a foundation through working the 12 Steps.

"More and more we find that the principles of the program guide our choices. The ability to choose wisely begins when we are able to be honest with ourselves about our motives and desires. Sometimes doing nothing is the most spiritual thing we can do. It can keep us from having to make amends later, and it gives us time to seek guidance from our Higher Power. We can have our feelings without being had by them. Laughter and joy can be as spiritual as prayer and service. Some say that enlightenment begins when we lighten up ourselves." -Living Clean (2012)

The 12 Steps

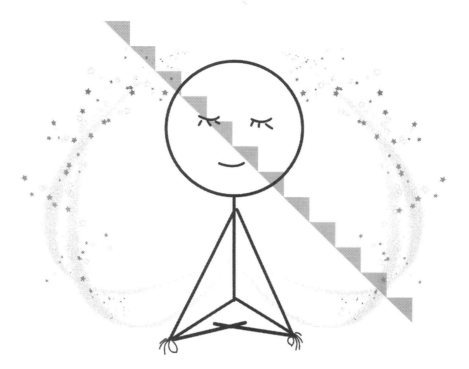

6

A Spirit of Collaboration

As a native of Southern California, I grew up traveling the complex freeway system in and around Los Angeles. I know this system well, which freeways travel north-south, or east-west, where they connect and split, how to get to the mountains, beach, or desert, and where the roads can take me in my daily life. I remember taking my first anatomy class in high school where my impression of the systems in the body were similar to my view of the roads and freeways. Main arteries and veins branch off into smaller arteries and veins, much like freeways, streets, and dirt roads branch off and become smaller the further away they get from the main hub. On the map I visualize the hub as downtown, where there is constant movement, freeways have movement in and out at all hours, and sometimes there is congestion. In the body I view the heart as the hub, as the constant flow of blood in and out keeps the system running, although sometimes we too get congested with things like stress, worry, anxiety, and fatigue. Many things are going on simultaneously, and driving varies from moving in ease and cooperation with surrounding cars, to busy clogs and being packed in tight traffic. This picture still holds true for me in the body too, as I see it in the layering of chakras, limbs, energy bodies, and steps. I view it as a sophisticated, choreography of movement and stagnation, with surprise obstacles thrown in every now and then to keep us aware and evolving.

"In relationship, these noble traditions (yoga, healing, 12 steps) *potentiate the possible and support the growth and recovery of the individual. In this age, we move beyond the need to divide and conquer, or blame and shame- others and ourselves."* - Gurucharan Khalsa PhD (2022)

First and foremost, both the 12 Steps and yoga, as written in the *Sutras*, are spiritual paths. They detail a spiritual, not religious, practice for balance, health, and happiness. The spirituality present in each path is not there for its own sake, it is to be accessed for the very practical application to heal and elevate the quality of life. We are invited to show up in our entirety in yoga and in the 12 Step fellowships, even our shadow side is welcome. We are free to drop the superficial mask and embrace our limitations as well as our strengths.

Similar threads between the 12 Step program and the yoga lifestyle are in the building of community and being of service to others. There is daily vigilance required to maintain abstinence, sobriety, and clean time. There is daily spiritual practice in yoga called *sadhana*.

Both systems rely on connection with community. In the program it's called fellowship. In yoga it's called *sangat*. Both the recovery and the yogic lifestyle provide guidelines for success. These are suggestions, not mandates. There is wiggle room and forgiveness along each path, but each is an entire system. Recovery is not a cafeteria line where we can have a little of this and a little of that, while entirely skipping what we think looks unappealing. The addict cannot afford to be finicky. If freedom is the goal, the path must be taken in its entirety, but don't worry there is no requirement for perfection. The system as a whole creates the magic of spirituality and the awareness of the Divine.

Manifestation or connection to the Divine is facilitated through the group. The steps begin with the word "we." This is not an individual program, but a we program, and the group or fellowship is essential for support and success. Similarly, in yoga we speak of consciousness as individual, group, and universal. Universal consciousness can only be obtained through the group, not solely by the individual.

The group is more powerful than the individual. In the program it is said something along the lines of; where two or three are gathered together, there you will find God. In yoga, a group is necessary for the practice in order to facilitate universal consciousness. We are all an expression of something larger than ourselves which we may refer to as Universe/ Source/Divine. Use whatever word you want, but group energy is key to personal growth.

"Rarely, if ever, are any of us healed in isolation. Healing is an act of communion." - Bell Hooks (2018)

Another function of community fellowship or *sangat* is to be of service to others. In the program it is said we can't keep what we have unless we give it away. Helping newer members find their place, and assisting other members in working the steps is a prescribed part of the recovery process. In yogic philosophy being of service to others is called *seva*, and it too is a recommended part of the spiritual lifestyle. What both the program and yogic lifestyle have figured out is that when one reaches out to help other people, the return reward is greater than the energy and time expended in helping others. When you stick your hand out to help another it can actually work to un-stick you. I have experienced this myself on my personal path of recovery, both in the aspect of group meditation and in giving away what was freely given to me in the spirit of helping the fellow addict.

"Service is a balm to both the spirit and the body." - Betty J. Eadie (1992)

All of the steps and all the limbs and bodies are given to us to help traverse life, but what really tests us and teaches us are relationships. Relationships are essential for us to glimpse our own inner world. Relationships mirror to us aspects we possess within ourselves. We may encounter qualities that we really like in others, as well as those we really dislike, or even despise. Believe it or not, this emotional and intellectual response to those seen as outside the self, provides the mirror that allows us to identify personal qualities we may want to keep, change, or eliminate. Bottom line is interpersonal relationships mirror what we like and don't like about ourselves. Your group doesn't need to be huge, but relationships are essential for personal progress.

There is a great little story about a grove of trees found in Nischala Joy Devi's book *The Secret Power of Yoga* that serves as a wonderful analogy.

"From the trunk upward, the trees appear to be independent, not connected to one another. However, if we venture several inches below the surface, we will find that these seemingly separate trees have their root systems intertwined. Their interdependency on one another for enduring strength and drawing in moisture unites them. Each is able to manifest a unique appearance while embracing the same consciousness."

We may have an individual human expression, but we need one another to in order to survive and to thrive.

Visualizing the intertwined root systems of trees, now let's look at how the chakras form a foundation for the layering and intertwining of 8 limbs, 10 bodies, and 12 Steps. The energy systems in the body are there waiting to serve us. The chakras and 10 bodies function automatically. They just go about their business of trying to keep us balanced and healthy, but ultimately take their cues by responding to the way we live our lives. The 8 limbs and 12 Steps are applied, not automatic, and can be used and integrated to direct energy. Intentional living affects the health of body, mind, and spirit. To create a personal change, the steps and limbs require a shift in attitude and new patterns of thought, followed by a change in behavior, and finally continued maintenance. Intentional changes in living affect the energy centers within and they respond to support our growth.

It's actually quite a simple program and simple process, however this does not mean it's easy. A simple program for complicated thinkers makes for an interesting trek. It's never about the destination, but the journey itself because that is where we live. We live, learn, and grow in the present moment. Living takes place within the journey. Let's remember to have some fun in recovery and enjoy the ride!

Principles of the 12 Steps

1. Honesty – A good, truthful look at the self
2. Hope – Connecting with belief that things can change
3. Faith – The idea of trusting in the recovery process, you're not in charge
4. Courage – Taking a deeper look at your behavior and feelings

5. Integrity – Being open to be accountable and heal
6. Willingness – A deeper dive into the truth of your own behavior
7. Humility – Neither inflate or deflate yourself, stand in the truth
8. Responsibility – Owning the harm you have caused
9. Discipline – Making amends means changing behavior
10. Perseverance – Continuing to monitor actions and attitude
11. Awareness – An openness to connect with higher guidance
12. Service – Helping others, walking like you talk

Principles of the Eight Limbs

1. Yama – Five Restraints; non-harming, truthfulness, non-stealing, moderation, non-possessiveness
2. Niyama – Five Disciplines; purity, contentment, courage, study, devotion
3. Asana - Posture
4. Pranayama -Breath Work
5. Pratyhar – Synchronization
6. Dharana - Concentration
7. Dyhana - Meditation
8. Samadhi – Absorption in Spirit

Principles/Attributes of the Chakras & The Ten Bodies

1. Foundation – A supportive starting place, connection to life
2. Sweetness – Going with the flow
3. Will of the Spiritual Warrior – Strength from the Divine
4. Unstruck – Purity of vibration
5. Purification – The clear human
6. Perception – Intuition
7. Infinite – Embracing the self beyond the identity of the body
8. Radiance – The light that shines from within

The first eight energy bodies correspond with the chakras in order. As with the chakras, their energetic reach is beyond their natural home in the body, they interact with each other and influence the whole body. Energy bodies nine and ten continue to interweave within and without the body and subtly permeate the universe.

When looking at the chakras, limbs, bodies, and steps all together, it brings me back to high school anatomy class where I can picture all the parts working together in a complicated, but harmonious flow. In our own lives we have the choice to create complication or harmony. I invite you to allow for the natural ebb and flow in the dance of your own life.

The Bigger Picture

Chakras, Limbs, Bodies, Steps

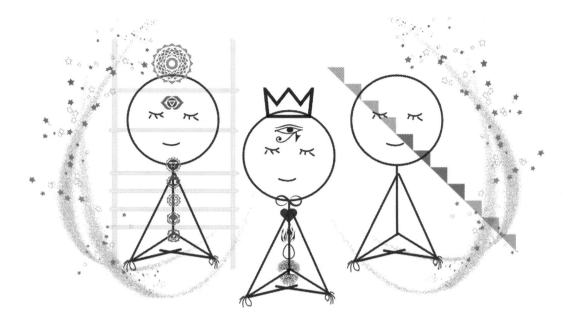

7

Introduction to Kundalini Yoga

The years I've spent in both recovery and in practicing yoga have made clear to me that the underlying spiritual principles weave together, complementing each other in a totally cohesive way. Before jumping into the steps and recommended yoga sets, I would like to share an introduction to Kundalini Yoga, which is the foundation for the yoga delivered herein. Some of the information in this chapter is taken from my previous book, *Yogable*, and condensed for the purpose of this book. If you can breathe, you can do yoga!

"The principles that underlie yoga are the principles that support a life of balance, flexibility, and vitality." - Dr. Deepak Chopra and Dr. David Simon (2004)

Kundalini yoga is known as the yoga of awareness, a precise technology of breath and movement in the body, which affect the mind and spirit. All forms of yoga actually tap into a reserve of Kundalini energy within the body, with the intent being energy integration. It works to clear, heal, and integrate the practitioner. Although the practice is precise, it is also very forgiving. I am a firm believer that the benefits of yoga are accessible to anyone and everyone. You do not need to have prior experience, be flexible, have a certain body type, or have any particular belief. Come as you are!

Yoga is a highly practical approach to the body and the mind, and as taught today, is for those of us who live within the realm of human society; we have families, friends, jobs, social engagements, and responsibilities to others. The yoga *kriyas* outlined in this book are a very direct application, tapping into the nervous system, stimulating the body on a glandular and cellular level. Have you ever felt like you are being run over by life, that time is moving too fast, or that you simply are not in control? The practice of yoga strengthens the nervous system so that the body and mind may more easily synchronize with the flow of life, with flexibility and resiliency, relieving feelings of being overwhelmed or being run over by a bulldozer. It works on the entire being through *pranayam* (breath), *asana* (posture), and meditation, which may include *mantra* (chanting) and *mudra* (hand positions), and deep relaxation.

The nervous system is stimulated and supported by yoga. Kundalini yoga increases circulation and energy moving throughout the body, improves both literal and energetic balance, decreases pain, helps to regenerate new brain cells, and increases connection between brain cells.

Yogic techniques are combined with an emphasis on coordinating breath and posture to create an experience. It's not about twisting yourself into a pretzel to attain a difficult posture in order to admire how great you look while practicing.

The focus of yoga is the experience - the benefits you receive in class and what carries over into your daily life. You may have heard that you can't save your face and your ass at the same time. Kundalini yoga helps to save your ass. It's about feeling good, not necessarily looking good. The coordination of breath and posture, meditation and relaxation, is what accounts for glandular stimulation and cleansing, which induces a feeling of renewal after practicing yoga. Simultaneously, muscle and tissue work to create strength and flexibility, while meditation works to cleanse the subconscious and direct the wavelengths of the brain. The combined effect of this work allows for a connection with the pulse of life and our personal divinity.

"Historically, it (yoga) was a tool to support us in living earthly life as a Spiritual Being." - *Hansa Knox*

The typical class outline observed for a Kundalini Yoga class:

Tune in with *Ong Namo, Guru Dev Namo*
Pranayam, or breath work
Warm-ups
Kriya, or exercise set
Deep Relaxation
Meditation
Sat Nam

Tuning-In

At the beginning of each class or personal practice, I recommend what is called "tuning-in" by chanting the words of the *Adi Mantra - Ong Namo, Guru Dev Namo*. In doing so, we are preparing for our experience, bowing to the Highest Consciousness as we call upon our own Divine Wisdom or inner teacher. The *Adi Mantra* connects us to the Divine Flow of Life, as well as the teachings and the teachers of past, present and future. Ultimately, we pause with reverence and chant to connect with the Divine Flow of Life. The mantra can be found on the companion soundtrack by Jap Dharam Rose, titled *8 Limbs, 10 Bodies, 12 steps: Yoga for Addiction Recovery* available on most popular streaming platforms.

It is worth noting that we are actually never disconnected from the Divine Flow of Life, we sometimes just get busy and forget that we are indeed connected.

This opening mantra is user friendly. When calling upon the Highest Consciousness, it is whatever each person believes and experiences. We do not bow to what someone else believes or what the teacher believes. We simply offer the mantra as we bow to a Universal Wisdom without intending to define it for others.

Om may be the familiar mantra for a hatha yoga practice. Both *Ong* and *Om* have a high vibrational quality. *Om* refers to the totality of Creation, and *Ong* refers to the Creating Force.

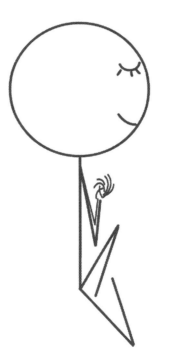

Traditionally tuning in is done while seated in Easy Pose with the hands in Prayer Pose. In Prayer Pose, the palms of the hands come together at the center of the chest, or heart center. The palms connect with light pressure and the thumbs rest on the sternum. The purpose of this posture is not actual prayer, but rather the calming effects the *mudra* (hand position) has on the body and mind. Prayer Pose helps to increase communication between the hemispheres of the brain, and supports balance and neutrality.

Resting in a neutral space for a few moments at the beginning of yoga class or personal practice allows for a peaceful transition from the demands and stresses of daily life to a mindful space. At the very least take a few deep breaths to clear the body and mind before moving into a yoga practice.

Breath or Pranayam

One of the first things we learn to do in yoga is breathe. You may be thinking, *"I've been breathing my whole life, I'm pretty sure I know how to breathe."* Perhaps, but what yoga initially does is open up the navel center, allowing breath to flow from the nose to below the navel. The breath creates an opening, a releasing of tightness or tension held within the inner recesses of the body, so that energy may move freely throughout the whole body. We learn to expand on the inhale and release, or contract, on the exhale. As we walk through life, many times we are not even aware when we are holding the breath, and thus stress, in the body. Yoga gives us the very basic awareness of proper breath.

The rate and intensity of the breath are fairly accurate indicators of one's emotional state. The breath is a powerful tool we can use to support and mold feelings of well-being – or not. So, the good news is that we can bring mindfulness to the breath in order to shift and uplift our mood and being. To reiterate from Chapters 3 and 4, breath work in yoga is called *pranayam,* and it refers to using the breath for basic energy management. Proper breath is the foundation for life, and the key to accessing both body and mind.

Breath work may be done as an intentional practice at the beginning of a class, after tuning in, or at the end of class in meditation. *Pranayam* is also practiced during yoga as the breath is linked to the posture. Two common breathing techniques in Kundalini yoga are Long Deep Breathing, as found in Chapter 4, and Breath of Fire as described below.

Breath of Fire

Breath of Fire is a rapid breath that closely resembles the panting of a dog. However, it is most often done through the nose. The breath is moved by a pumping or pulsing movement of the navel and solar plexus area. The diaphragm remains relaxed as it moves with the breath. On the inhale the belly is relaxed, and on the exhale the navel point/ solar plexus contracts, pulling in toward the spine, pressing the diaphragm up so that all of the air is expelled from the lungs. The inhale and exhale are equal in duration; if you focus on the exhale, the inhale will take care of itself because your body wants to breathe. Breath of Fire is a diaphragmatic breath. Breath of Fire is fast and powerful, cleansing and energizing, and it does build heat within the body. Start slowly at 40 to 60 breaths per minute. The breath can be built up to 2-3 breaths per second.

Of course, Breath of Fire can be done at a slower pace, so slow down if needed. If you start to feel dizzy take a break and return to a natural breath. I invite new students to place one hand on the belly to be sure that the contraction happens on the exhale as the body becomes accustomed to the practice of Breath of Fire. While this practice may feel awkward at first, it will soon become second nature.

It is interesting to note that some traditions refer to this practice as skull cleansing breath. Sign me up, please! I still have days where I feel like my brain could benefit from a good scrubbing.

Benefits of Breath of Fire

- Oxygenates and purifies the body
- Releases toxins and deposits from the lungs, mucous linings, and blood vessels
- Expands lung capacity and increases vital strength
- Strengthens the entire nervous system, all seventy-two thousand nerves
- Restores balance between the sympathetic and parasympathetic nervous systems
- Strengthens the navel
- Increases physical endurance and prepares one to act effectively
- Helps to reduce addictive tendencies, thoughts, and impulses
- Promotes a positive neutrality in the mind
- Increases oxygen delivery to the brain
- Boosts immune system function
- Insulates the nerves, providing for a type of life force cushion
- Calms the disposition and combats stress
- With regular practice, Breath of Fire helps to ease temper tantrums and angry outbursts

<u>Breath of Fire in Ego Eradicator posture</u>

Sit in Easy Pose, or your easy seat of choice. Extend the arms up at a 60 degree angle, like the letter V, with the fingers curled into the pads of the palms and the thumbs extended out. Thumbs wills stretch upward as though plugged into the universe. Close your eyes gently and concentrate above the head as you practice Breath of Fire.

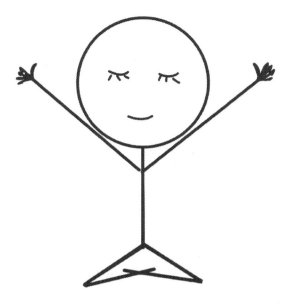

Breath of Fire is contraindicated for those who are:

- Women in the first few days of their menstrual cycle
- Experiencing diaphragm or rib injuries
- Currently experiencing or are predisposed to pelvic organ prolapse
- Pregnant
- Experiencing pain with the breath
- Children

Warm-Ups

Although warm-ups are not a required element of yoga, they can be quite beneficial in preparing for a yoga *kriya*, allowing the body to not only stretch, but also settle into a seated posture offering increased comfort and a sense of grounding. Typically, if warm-ups are used, only a few are suggested prior to practicing a *kriya*. A complete warm-up set can be found at the end of this chapter. The set may be done in its entirety or you may choose a few of the warm-up exercise options to stretch and to open the flow of energy to the spine, hips, legs and shoulders, which increases flexibility and circulation throughout the whole body.

What is a *Kriya*?

A *kriya* is a sequence of prescribed yoga postures or an exercise set which may also include breath work and meditation. It is considered a complete action. Unless otherwise noted, the *kriyas* herein are given as originally taught in the Kundalini yoga tradition by Yogi

Bhajan. *Pranayam*, *Kriya*, or meditations will be suggested for each of the 12 Steps in following chapters.

The *kriyas* are taught as given, and in addition to working on all of the energy centers in the body, they target different areas of the human psyche, including body, mind, and emotion. For the purpose of making the *kriyas* accessible to all, I have published a previous book titled *"Yogable, A Gentle Approach to Yoga for Special Populations"* wherein I give modifications and choices alongside the original set of directions for the yoga postures. Should you desire a gentle practice I recommend consulting the aforementioned book. I do share some adaptations for the yoga within this book, and always encourage you to listen to your own body and to participate in yoga to your own ability. There is no competition and no finish line to cross.

The point of yoga is the experience, not perfecting posture. This practice, although sometimes out of the box and seemingly strange, is the perfect antidote to the mundane human condition because it is all about encouraging you to achieve your full potential. Kundalini yoga is actually a precise application of technology that accommodates all levels and abilities. It is compassionate in the sense that you start where you are and honor your body. It wakes the body up from the inside out, and makes you feel good. Moving the body aids the subconscious in letting go of old ideas, patterns, and experiences.

That being said, the process itself may not always be warm and fuzzy. You may love some of the exercises, and others may push your buttons. I don't share this to be disheartening or as a warning, but the reality is in any area of life work is required to achieve amazing results. The type of work I'm referring to in both yoga and recovery can include honesty, commitment, effort, being present, being intentional, and simply showing up. I'll let you in on a little secret - 75% of the work is just showing up. Once we've shown up, we only have to apply the remaining 25% to get the full benefit. Now this 25% may sometimes feel like a warm breeze or soft caress, and other times may feel like course grade sandpaper rubbing on the skin.

The grit of sandpaper needed is determined by the project at hand. For instance, in a woodworking project, the piece of lumber starts out raw, possibly bumpy and rough. The carpenter would need to begin to tame the unfinished log with a lower grit sand paper. Once the project becomes smoother and more manageable, a higher grit paper may be substituted, increasing the grit slowly, to achieve a seamless polish. People entering the recovery process are typically pretty rough, not unlike a newly felled log. The practice of yoga and meditation may feel, at times, like harsh, scratchy sandpaper, but as we begin to smooth out our rough edges the sandpaper feels less gritty too. Since recovery is a continual journey, there is no destination; our yoga practice and the refining effect of the sandpaper changes with us, adjusting grit to take care of any bumps, bruises, or splinters we may encounter along the way. In this analogy the sandpaper is the practice of yoga and especially meditation.

I think my favorite story from teaching in treatment centers, which pretty much sums up the practice of Kundalini yoga, came in the form of a quiet whisper in the back of the room. For those of you who are familiar with Kundalini yoga you'll know we do different and interesting *kriyas* and meditations; sometimes they could even be described as weird. Let me remind you that the practice is all about how it makes you feel, not how you look. Anyway, I was in a treatment center for male parolees teaching yoga to a pretty mellow, compliant class, and in the back row there was a small group of tough looking men. Now, I can hear very well, and when what was meant to be a whispered comment reached my ears, I had to refrain from laughing aloud. One of the men, a gang member fresh out of prison, with tattoos covering his bald head and his entire face, leaned over to his friend and said in regard to the yoga practice, "*Man, this is the craziest shit I've ever seen, and I thought I'd seen everything.*" I went on teaching class and never let him know I heard his comment, but thought to myself, "*you just got out of prison and your face is covered in tattoos, and this is the craziest shit you've ever seen?!*" I believe his statement to be true.

Deep Relaxation

Upon concluding a *kriya,* there is typically a period of deep relaxation (*savasana*) practiced while lying on the back to allow for the assimilation of the yoga prior to meditation. This is not optional or unimportant. The body requires about 10 minutes of active deep relaxation (not a nap) daily in order to function at its best. Relaxation after the *kriya* can last anywhere from 3 to 11 minutes. Sometimes the meditation is included in the *kriya,* and deep relaxation follows, but meditation is usually practiced after relaxation. Wherever deep relaxation may fall in the structure of the practice it is important to find a comfortable posture lying on the back with the arms and legs away from the torso, palms facing up with relaxed fingers, and feet dropping slightly out to the side. This posture is called Corpse Pose. Any discomfort experienced in the lower back while the legs are extended along the ground may be alleviated by bending the knees and keeping the feet flat on the floor. Upon exiting the period of *savasana* a wake-up routine is helpful in coming back to awareness and the physical body, providing movement in a way that allows one to come back to the present slowly and safely.

In Kundalini yoga we move out of deep relaxation by bringing awareness back to the body and breath, then wiggle the fingers and toes, rotate the wrists and ankles, rub the palms and the soles of the feet together, and lastly bring the knees into the chest and rock the body up and down along the spine a few times before rocking all the way back up into Easy Pose.

Meditation

Meditation may come before or after deep relaxation. It is a crucial part of the practice of yoga. Meditation helps to develop a neutral mind (also called the meditative mind), focus, concentration, awareness, clarity, calming, stability and an overall sense of well-being. Meditation is really a detoxification of the subconscious, a practice to clean out the mental garbage that weighs us down. With regular practice the actual aim of yoga and meditation is to direct the waves of the mind, with the idea being that the mind is a servant to the soul, not the other way around. It's an invitation to open the door to re-discover what lies underneath the outer facade.

It is a common myth that meditation is always supposed to be a calm, peaceful, soothing practice where one quiets the mind and rests in stillness. Have you tried to tell the mind to be quiet on demand lately? It can be like trying to stop the sun from shining or the rain from falling. The job of the mind is to move; it is ever in motion. This is not to say that we can't find a still, quiet, peaceful place within, but don't worry if it doesn't happen spontaneously and naturally. As stated, meditation is like detox for the subconscious, a clearing out of all the emotions, traumas, and actions we've stored that are not in our immediate consciousness. This meditative process is not always comfy and cozy. It can actually be quite loud and uncomfortable, and it may include anger tears as it releases our pain and brings us closer to our true self. I'm really not trying to talk you out of practicing meditation, but letting you know it's serious work with serious benefits. Ultimately the practice of meditation begins to feel like coming home, and it very well may feel comfortable and serene.

The effects of meditation deepen with extended practice, both in number of days, and minutes practiced. Below you can find what to expect with regard to days and times spent in meditation.

Days of Meditation:

40 days to break a habit
90 days to create a new habit
120 days to make that habit yours, to own it
1,000 days to master the new habit

Off topic of meditation, but in line with creating new habits, we can use this information when cultivating simple daily structure that we want to make stick. Today my son asked me how many days in a row he has to make his bed in the morning (this has been an area of contention between us for years) for it to become an automatic habit. I suggested he start with today and then aim for 40 days. Keep it simple.

Minutes of Meditation:

3 minutes – taps into the electromagnetic field and the blood
11 minutes – begins to change nerves and the glandular system
22 minutes – balances the negative, positive, and neutral minds for cohesion
31 minutes – affects all of the cells and the rhythms of the body
62 minutes – affects gray matter in the brain

As you can see, it takes more than one session of meditation to truly reap the rewards. In addition to benefits already mentioned, meditation also increases efficiency, and helps to release unhealthy patterns. If you want to accelerate the effect of the aforementioned sandpaper, spend more time in meditation.

One of the things I initially loved about Kundalini yoga is that many of the meditations are active, meaning they include *mudra* (hand positions), movement, and *mantra* (chanting) with precise instructions. I didn't have to sit down and try to force my mind to be quiet by willpower alone. Finally, I had found a method to access the still, quiet space within through the use of body and voice, movement and sound vibration. For proper rhythm and pronunciation, the meditations with mantra given in this book are available for streaming on the soundtrack titled *8 Limbs, 10 Bodies, 12 Steps: Yoga for Addiction Recovery* by Jap Dharam Rose.

Closing the practice

The session is ended by chanting a *Sat Nam*. This provides closure with reverence and a sense of grounding. The *Sat* is a long vibration, followed by a short, soft *Nam*. *Sat Nam* is a mantra to honor truth as identity for all. *Namaste* would be the familiar closing mantra for a *Hatha* practice, honoring the spirit in all. Both of these mantras are typically accompanied by a seated forward bow.

Student Reported Benefits of Yoga

- Improved balance
- More energy throughout the day

- Decreased stress
- Increased relaxation
- Decreased pain in the physical body
- Improved sleep
- Increased sense of self-worth
- Improved attitude and outlook on life
- Better quality of breath
- Increased flexibility in body and mind
- Improved digestion
- Clearer thinking
- A sense of increased mental well-being
- Increased creativity
- Decreased anxiety
- Less reactive and self-destructive
- Better emotional regulation
- Increased feelings of connection with body and mind
- Increased passion, joy, and honesty

Additional Yoga Terms

Prana

Prana with a capital "P" is found in five different frequencies within the body. It is the first unit of energy that interpenetrates every atom in the body and the entirety of creation. Two of these frequencies found in the body are *prana*, with a lower case "p", and *apana*. These frequencies are present in the *Prana* of the ten bodies. It's the *prana* with a small 'p' that yoga most often refers to in classes.

The simplest translation of *prana*, with the lowercase "p", is "life force." The life force of *prana* is what we bring into the body and it coordinates the energies of the body and mind. It unites intelligence and matter. The natural home for *prana* in the body is in the area of the heart, chest and neck, and it is linked to respiration. It is not the breath itself, but *prana* has a special relationship with the breath, as breath circulates *prana*, and *prana* stimulates the systems of the body. *Prana* is expansive, inspiring, and prepares one to engage in life.

Apana

Apana is the eliminating force or energy in the body. It resides in the lower abdominal area, and quite literally governs our physical elimination and release of toxins. Energetically *apana* regulates what we need to let go of and what we need to keep. Too much accumulated *apana* in the body may manifest as feeling slow, heavy, lazy, or mentally foggy.

Through the practice of Kundalini yoga *kriyas*, both the life force of *prana* and the eliminating force of *apana* are stimulated within the body. They accumulate and meet at the navel point to stimulate the Kundalini energy, which supports an even energy exchange of inflow and outflow. This blending helps to increase a balanced emotional and intellectual response to the external environment and regulate the individual mood.

Mantra

Man translates as mind, and *Trang* translates as a wave or projection. *Mantra* typically translates as chanting, and is a projection of the mind through sound vibration. Chanting during meditation is a conscious practice to tame and direct the mind. The elements that make *mantra* effective are rhythm, projecting from the navel, and pronunciation. *Mantra* is effective, positive vibration of sound.

Mudra

A *mudra* is a hand position in which pressure is applied between fingers, palms, or specific parts of the hand to create a seal. The seal is a special pressure that communicates a flow of energy to the corresponding part of the body or brain. Each *mudra* elicits a unique response, as found in Chapter 2.

Bandhas/Body Locks

Venus Lock

Venus Lock is a component found in the yoga sets presented in this book, and is referred to frequently in the practice of Kundalini yoga. Venus Lock is an interlacing of the fingers while bringing the palms of the hands together. Traditionally it was taught that women interlace with the left thumb on top, so that it is in the outermost position, and men interlace in the opposite way, with the right thumb on the outside. Left stimulates the feminine energy, which is cooling and calming, and the right stimulates the masculine energy, which is warming and energizing. It is appropriate to encourage each student to choose their Venus Lock based on whether they want to work with the Divine Feminine energy or the Divine Masculine energy, depending on current needs and mood.

Toe Lock

Although technically not a lock, the toe hold used in forward folds is a technique that is sometimes referred to as the toe lock. If the seated forward fold affords the opportunity to reach the toes, it is recommended to take the index and middle finger and wrap them around the back of the big toe, while gently pressing on the toenail with the thumb. The ring finger and pinky tuck in toward the palm. This gentle pressure point provides a grounding point for the fold and stimulates the pituitary gland.

Mulbandh

The *Mulbandh* or Root Lock can be used in a variety of yoga postures. It can be applied on a suspended inhale or exhale. The Root Lock is applied by contracting the muscles of the rectum, sex organs and navel point with a gentle upward pull. Energy is directed up along the spinal column for integration. This moves in line with the natural flow of energy in the body.

Applying a gentle Root Lock will help to create a stable internal foundation for most seated postures, especially during meditation. This gentle, or light pull of the Root Lock also helps provide support for the spine and improves posture.

Jalandhar Bandh

Jalandhar Bandh or Neck Lock is applied as directed when the spine is straight, as in a seated posture. The Neck Lock is applied by simultaneously lengthening the back of the neck and pulling the chin slightly in and back, but not up or down. The head stays in a neutral position and the chest remains up and open. This lock lifts the heart, provides focus, stabilization, and proper flow both physically and energetically between the head and the body.

Body locks work much like breath in the sense that they are tools for directing energy in the body. Two more locks that are worth mentioning, are *Uddiyana Bandh* which is the Diaphragm Lock and *Maha Bandh* which refers to applying all the body locks at the same time to create the Great Lock.

Practical Application: Steps & Yoga Sets

The yoga sets are given as taught, and I've added only a few adapted choices for some of the postures. You are responsible for your own body. In yoga it is your job to honor your body by engaging in the practice at a level that is right for you.

Prior to beginning the chapters on steps and yoga, I want to make a note about a very special exercise/meditation called *Sat Kriya*. It is found within three of the yoga sets given, and you will find the directions for *Sat Kriya* explained in three different ways, each highlighting a slightly different focus, but each building and adding to the description prior. *Sat Kriya* is also known as a stand-alone *kriya,* meaning done on its own it is a complete action. You can practice this all by itself, outside of the actual yoga set, with amazing results. Be sure to relax after practicing for at least as long as the duration of the meditation. It is versatile in that it functions as an exercise and/or a meditation. The mantra used is *"Sat Nam"* and it means "truth is my identity." It is no coincidence that it shows up in so many of the yoga sets I have chosen for addiction recovery. It is packed with the power of manifestation and creative transformation.

Before practicing a yoga *kriya, pranayam,* or meditation, please tune in and center yourself by chanting *"Ong Namo, Guru Dev Namo"* three times. An alternate suggestion, given earlier in this chapter, may also be used to enter your practice in a peaceful manner.

As we move into the steps and yoga sets, it is not my intention to give definitive instruction on working the 12 Steps, nor to replace or substitute information on the steps found in recovery literature. As I write on the steps, I will be sharing information based on my personal experience, along with concepts and ideas that I have found helpful in the course of my recovery and yoga practice spanning over three decades. Please take what you can use, and feel free to leave the rest.

The following chapters speak to each of the twelve steps and share narratives of personal experience, tips for application, testimonials, a bonus activities or recipes, along with yoga recommendations, to include *kriya, pranayam,* and meditation. The chapters on the steps reference those in the recovery process, but are intended to also be educational for yoga teachers, therapists, and other professionals, as well as family and friends of the recovering person.

Warm-Up Exercise Set

This is a fabulous set for warming up and stretching the body that can be done prior to other yoga sets and meditations found later in this book. This is not an actual *kriya,* but a complete warm-up set that can be referred to and practiced again and again. To begin exercise times can be shortened to 1 minute each, slowly building to 2 to 3 minutes if desired. Take care of knees with alternate seated postures if needed, such as Easy Pose or sitting in a chair.

The series of forward folds, or Life Nerve Stretches, exercises 6 and 7 may be modified by only folding forward to tolerance. Rather than aiming for the feet, let the hands slide down the legs and hold where there is a gentle challenge, perhaps knees, shins, or ankles. A yoga strap may also be used in forward folds to provide support.

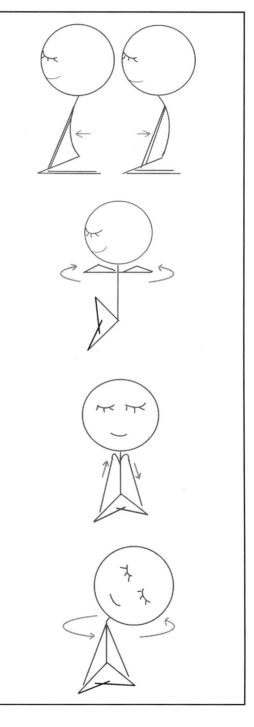

1. Spinal Flex. Sitting on the heels, flex the spine back and forth, inhaling as it arches forward, exhaling as the spine contracts back. Continue for 2-3 minutes.

2. Spinal Twist. Sitting on the heels, with hands on the shoulders, fingers in front, thumbs in back, twist spine side to side for 2-3 minutes.

3. Shoulder Shrugs. Relax hands down on Knees, and inhale raising shoulders up to ears, exhale relaxing them down. Repeat for 2-3 minutes.

4. Neck Rolls. Tilt the chin down to the chest and gently circle the head, breathing slowly and deeply, keeping the shoulders relaxed. Make slow, smooth circles, ironing out any kinks as you go. Continue for 1-2 minutes, reverse for another 1-2 minutes.

5. Cat Cow Pose. Come onto the hands and knees. The hands are shoulder-width apart with the fingers facing forward. The knees are directly below the hips. Inhale and tilt the pelvis forward, arching the spine down, and stretching the head and neck back. Then exhale and tilt the pelvis the opposite way, arching the spine up and bring the chin to the chest. Continue for 2-3 minutes.

6. Life Nerve Stretches:

   a. Both legs stretched out in front, bend at the hips and grab toes. Exhale as you fold forward and the head comes down toward the knees, rise up as you inhale, head following. Continue moving up and down for 1-2 minutes.

   b. Legs stretched out in front, bend the left knee and place the left heel in the right thigh, and repeat inhaling up and exhaling down over the leg for 1-2 minutes. Switch legs and repeat for 1-2 minutes.

7. Wide Leg Forward Fold. Stretch legs out in front and then stretch them out wide. Fold forward and hold on to the toes. Inhale up, and exhale down to alternate knees. Continue for 1-2 minutes.

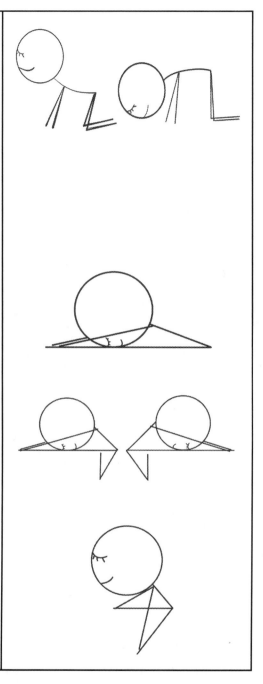

8

Step One

"We admitted that we were powerless over our addiction, that our lives had become unmanageable."

"Forgive yourself for not being at peace. The moment you completely accept your non-peace, your non-peace is transmuted into peace. Anything you accept fully will get you there, will take you to peace. This is the miracle of surrender." -Eckhart Tolle (1999)

What do you mean I'm powerless over a beer? You mean I can't learn how to drink like a lady and shoot dope on the weekend? You mean, we don't ever use drugs, we abstain completely? This last concept flew right over my head when I was new, as I could not comprehend this idea. I did, however, completely comprehend that my life was unmanageable and I could not stop using. But how was admitting and accepting my addiction going to help me not use drugs?

First and foremost, an awareness that there is a problem is needed before any change can commence. The negative experience of hitting a dark bottom may be a catalyst for change, or an agent for motivation. This step is where the addicted individual can stop running from their own feelings and story. An honest look at personal problems due to addiction may help in developing needed awareness. Truth destroys illusions. Whether illusions have been built for the purpose of denial, protection, or fantasy, truth breaks the spell. From here the addict can begin to break out of old patterns of thinking and behaving, and move toward an acceptance of Step One and one's own powerlessness and unmanageability.

Personally, it took me time to learn about acceptance; what is it, what does it really mean, how can it benefit me? To accept is to acknowledge the truth, to look at things as they really are, instead of how we want them to be. Well, for most addicts taking a long, hard look at the reality of the consequences experienced from active addiction is a painful road to walk. Denial is a tool used to continue on the path of destruction through excuses, justification, or ignoring problems. Step One strips the denial away, so the addict may see clearly. When we step into the light of truth we can stop fighting and admit to ourselves and others that our way is not working. The acceptance of the disease of addiction is not something that can be done on an intellectual level if recovery is to be maintained. Acceptance of addiction needs to reach down to the depths of the spirit, radiating through every cell in the body, casting no doubt that there is not a way to safely engage in the addiction of choice. A thorough First Step helps to identify and release reservations. It is an inner knowing that trying to fight the addiction is futile. Hence, we find the solution of acceptance and surrender and we stop struggling.

Admitting defeat may induce anxiety as the unknown can be uncomfortable. I invite you to sit with the discomfort of uncertainty. Uncertainty implies that there is no particular outcome to rely on and no definite answers waiting on the other end. However, when we stop fervently trying to work another angle, or try out another plan, and simply come to rest in the unknown, we open ourselves to trusting in the universal wisdom of uncertainty and our own intuition. Stepping out of the comfort zone is a must for personal growth. Letting go of the need to know all outcomes, opens the way to inner peace and new possibilities. This is a passive, positive action of surrendering.

Personally, I had to admit that no matter what I tried in the past, on my own I could not control my using. To make peace with being powerless over a single beer I had to look at my history. When in my life had I ever enjoyed one single beer? Never, not even as a young teen. I was able to see that perceived control in any area of life was false. This illusion of control is what keeps many of us stuck on the merry-go-round for years. I had to take a look at my thinking, and it may sound silly, but a simple story from my waitressing days shed light on the fact that I don't even think like a non-addict.

I worked in a Mexican food restaurant for years, and sometimes I covered a cocktail lounge shift and worked in the bar. I never understood why people would order a drink, sip on it, and leave half in the glass. Seriously this made absolutely no sense to me. Only one margarita? To this day, it doesn't resonate with me. I used to think, what is wrong with them? First of all, why would you only have one, and if you did order a second, why would you leave any behind in the glass or bottle? If you don't ever want only one, then my dear, you may be an addict.

Taking away the drugs or the addiction of choice only eliminates the identified problem. Step One brings us to the realization that we are the problem, not the identified addiction. The real problem lies within our thinking and the way we respond to our inner and outer world. The behavior is only the external symptom.

The unmanageability in my case was obvious. I was a mess. Who knew admitting the mess I made of my life was going to actually be a positive step toward getting into the solution? That is the power of taking an honest appraisal. For those who can maintain outward appearances, the unmanageability may be uncovered by looking inward to the emotional or mental state of being.

As soon as defeat, in the positive sense of the word, is accepted we are empowered by choice. As long as we think we've got it under control we're fighting a losing battle. In fact, fighting addiction at all is pointless. Once we surrender our attempt to control, we are given the power to choose. This may sound paradoxical, but it's true that surrender is actually empowering. What we come to see is that control is not possible. Before I worked the First Step, I did not have the choice to use or not. I simply used. Step One gives us a choice and opens the door to making new decisions. For many it is a relief to know addiction is a real problem, not a moral deficiency, and that there is a solution. The next hurdle for some to overcome is that there is no quick fix, that recovery takes honest work and continued action.

Returning to the concept of acceptance, it is with honesty we are able to apply this step in all areas of life: self, other people, places, and things. We may possibly begin with tolerance, simply tolerating circumstances around us without acting out in selfish or aggressive ways. Tolerance is a stepping stone to acceptance. We are not asked to live our lives as doormats teetering on the edge of tolerance, rather we are encouraged to go further within to experience true acceptance. The best thing I ever heard about step one is that the level of our acceptance is directly proportionate to the level of our serenity. This one statement allowed me to see what was in it for me, answering the "why" behind practicing honesty and acceptance. At the time, I wasn't really sure what serenity felt like, but it sounded good. Integrating the acceptance of powerlessness comes in handy as the years go by because being powerless and practicing acceptance is not only applied to addiction. It permeates every nook and cranny of life. If you really think you have the ability to control things, try stopping a bad case of diarrhea with your will power.

I am hard pressed to give an example of what in this world we may actually have control over, and thus, I prefer using the word command. Now that we know we're the problem and we have taken the First Step, we do actually have the power of command over the way we react and respond to life around us. I have a special needs son who has been challenging since day one. He's an adult now, but when he was only eight years old, he began having seizures; grand mal, stop breathing, turn blue kind of seizures. The most powerless I have ever felt in my life was watching my child convulse violently, stop breathing, and turn blue in front of my eyes, and not being able to do one single thing to help stop the convulsions or to make him breathe again. I was however, able to stay in command of my behavior, be present, pray harder than ever before, and be humbled into a new level of acceptance.

Time gives experience in living life on life's terms, and the steps give us the tools to rise to the occasion.

An added gift of the principle of acceptance is that we are able to let go of our expectations and judgement about others and their path. When we let go of our need to manage and control events and other people, we find a new inner peace. If you're new and this sounds like a load of BS, let curiosity drive you to take a closer look at surrender and acceptance as an answer to personal suffering.

Inner peace is actually a natural response to authentic acceptance. Active addition is an expression of non-peace. Through taking an honest look at our lives, including the physical, mental, emotional, and spiritual realms, and accepting life as it is, not as we want it to be, we are able to begin to take responsibility for our behavior. It is only through taking responsibility for our addiction that we gain any freedom. One of the first limbs of yoga also teaches us to create the foundation of an honest lifestyle, and that our freedom comes from accountability.

"And acceptance is the answer to all my problems today. When I am disturbed, it is because I find some person, place, thing, or situation — some fact of my life — unacceptable to me, and I can find no serenity until I accept that person, place, thinking, or situation as being exactly the way it is supposed to be at this moment. Nothing, absolutely nothing happens in God's world by mistake. Until I could accept my alcoholism, I could not stay sober; unless I accept life completely on life's terms, I cannot be happy. I need to concentrate not so much on what needs to be changed in the world as on what needs to be changed in me and in my attitudes." – Alcoholics Anonymous (1939)

When I was beginning to jot down ideas for this book, I kept a notebook on my nightstand to write down middle of the night inspirations. I was awakened one morning to this statement given specifically in relation to Step One. Although I have not heard it shared in meetings that I am aware of, it has stayed with me ever since I woke from the dream. It was not a soft, subtle message, but a loud, in--your-face message. As I share it now, Step One is an invitation to *"Wake up and fall in love with life!"*

Testimonial:

"Kundalini yoga sets, meditations, and the overall lifestyle of being a Kundalini practitioner makes it easy to recognize when I'm in denial about my addictive behaviors, my health issues, and to recognize the truth about difficult and dysfunctional relationships. Consequently, my practice enables me to get into acceptance, surrender, and serenity much more quickly

than my self-will run riot. Resentments and self-pity slip away in the face of recognizing that the other person IS me. Ultimately, through Kundalini yoga, I've learned to intuitively and energetically recognize and realize my own divine power and how to remain true to this new way of living." -Jaskamal Kaur

Bonus:

Nutritional Juice Recipe

Grapefruit, Apple and Carrot Juice
A wonderful detoxification drink. Very cleansing as well as an energy boost.
                    -Mukta Kaur Khalsa, Ph.D., *Meditations for Addictive Behavior (2008)*

Combine 1/3 cup grapefruit juice, 1/3 cup apple juice and 1/3 cup carrot juice, for a total of 8 ounces. It is best to use fresh, organic juices.

Yoga Recommendation:

Step One begins with the very basic foundation of recovery. Basic Spinal Energy Series set works on the first chakra, addressing fears and insecurities to support balance in the earth element. It is grounding and helps to integrate energy.

Take a few moments to write on your thoughts and feelings about powerlessness and unmanageability:

Basic Spinal Energy Series

Age is measured by the flexibility of the spine: to stay young, stay flexible. This series works systematically from the base of the spine to the top. All 26 vertebrae receive stimulation and all the chakras receive a burst of energy. This makes it a good series to do before meditation. Many people report greater mental clarity after regular practice of this kriya. A contributing factor is the increased circulation of the spinal fluid, which is crucially linked to having a good memory. If you are a beginner, you can reduce the times and the number of repetitions. The rests between exercises can also be increased.

1. Spinal Flex. Sit in Easy Pose. Grab the ankles with both hands and deeply inhale. Flex the spine forward and lift the chest up. On the exhale, flex the spine backwards. Keep the head level so it does not "flip-flop." Repeat 108 times. Rest 1 minute. Spinal flex greatly alters the proportions and strengths of alpha, theta, and delta waves.

2. Spinal Flex. Sit on the heels in Rock Pose. Place the hands flat on the thighs. Flex spine forward with the inhale, backward with the exhale. Mentally vibrate Sat on the inhale, Nam on the exhale. Repeat 108 times. Rest 2 minutes.

3. Spinal Twist. In Easy Pose, grasp the shoulders with fingers in front, thumbs in back. Inhale and twist to the left, exhale and twist to the right. Continue 26 times and inhale facing forward. Rest 1 minute.

4. Bear Grip. Curl the fingers of each hand and lock them together at the heart center. Move the elbows in a see-saw motion, inhaling as the left elbow comes up and exhaling as the right elbow comes up. Continue 26 times and inhale, exhale, pull the Root Lock. Relax 30 seconds.

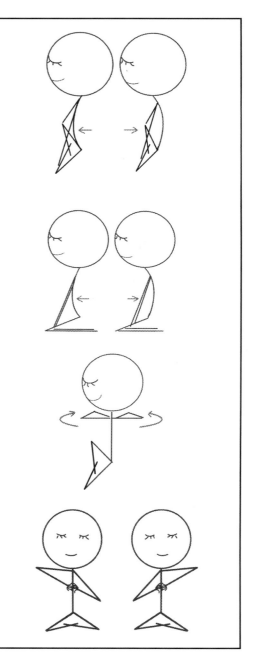

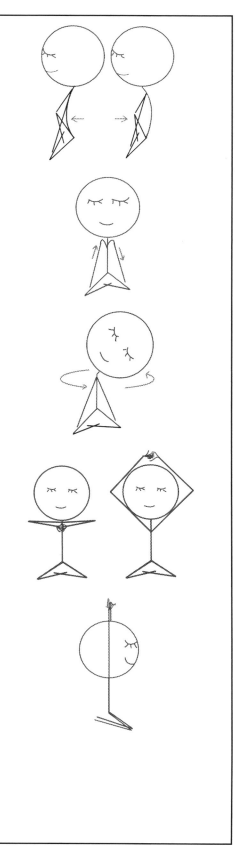

5. Spinal Flex. In Easy Pose, grasp the knees firmly. Keeping the elbows straight, begin to flex the upper spine. Inhale forward, exhale back. Repeat 108 times. Rest 1 minute.

6. Shoulder Shrugs. Shrug both shoulders up on the inhale, down on the exhale. Do this for 1 to 2 minutes. Inhale and hold 15 seconds with shoulders pressed up. Relax the shoulders.

7. Neck Rolls. Roll the neck slowly to the right 5 times, then to the left 5 times. Inhale, and bring the neck straight.

8. Bear Grip. Lock the fingers in Bear Grip at the throat level. Inhale – apply the Root Lock. Exhale – apply the Root Lock. Then raise the hands above the top of the head. Inhale – apply Root Lock. Exhale – apply Root Lock. Repeat the cycle 2 more times.

9. Sat Kriya. Sit on the heels with the arms overhead and the palms together. Interlace the fingers except for the index fingers, which point straight up. Men cross the right thumb over the left: women cross the left thumb over the right. Chant *Sat* and pull the navel point in: chant *Naam* and relax it. Continue powerfully with a steady rhythm for at least 3 minutes, then inhale, apply Root Lock and squeeze the energy from the base of the spine to the top of the skull. Exhale, hold the breath out and apply all the locks. Inhale and relax.

| 10. Relax completely on your back for 15 minutes.

A description of the body locks is included in Chapter 7. | 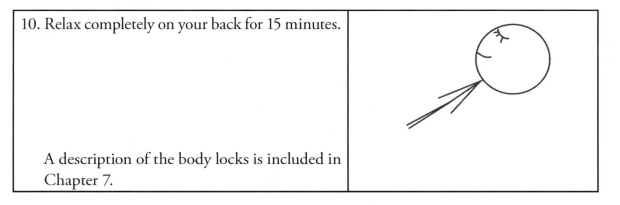 |

9

Step Two

"We came to believe that a Power Greater than ourselves could restore us to sanity."

"Although many drug users thought of Kundalini Yoga as another way to get "high," Kundalini Yoga is a way to becoming the higher self. It is getting out of pain, subconscious turmoil, and boredom. It gives you energy from within that cannot be given or created by any outside substance." -Shakti Parwha Kaur Khalsa (1996)

Wait, what, now I'm insane? The need to be restored to sanity implies insanity. Well, if insanity is defined as doing the same thing over and over and expecting different results, then yes, put me on the list. I was always going to begin kicking my habit on a Monday, then I'd use on Monday, and have to wait until the following Monday. Don't ask me why it had to be a Monday, but it made perfect sense to me, and that perfect Monday never came. The insane part is despite evidence to the contrary week after week, I always believed it was going to be next Monday that I would begin to get my life together.

Add in the honest look taken at the self in Step One, and it's difficult to try to justify addiction as sane behavior. Now, in Step Two we connect with a Power Greater than ourselves for help in restoring us to sanity. If you look up restoration in the dictionary it depicts a return to the original state.

Yoga teaches that our original state is joy, love, truth, and clarity. Many addicts report that they have never experienced this state of true, divine being, and mostly likely none of us remember this state from birth. So, it is here we can ask ourselves what type of restoration we desire. We may simply desire to be

restored to our pre-addiction state. When this degree of restoration happens, we may realize we are still the same person minus the drugs or behaviors, and we are still dissatisfied within our own skin. Working the steps in recovery, we have the opportunity to be restored on a more profound level, beyond the surface of simply not using, to a state of healing and grace. To be clear, this is a process, not typically an event, and we get to choose how much we want to grow.

First, the addict is asked to come to believe that it is possible to recover, and that there is a Power Greater than the self to help along the way. Addicts usually don't just wake up one morning bubbling with belief. For me personally, belief came from listening and connecting to other addicts. In the rooms of 12 Step programs, I heard people speaking about the way I felt, and I knew I had found a place I belonged. I had never heard people openly share about the kind of insecurities, resentments, and fear that I lived with until I claimed a seat in 12 Step meetings. Not only were people overcoming paralyzing emotions, they were moving beyond maladaptive behavior as well. I was so relieved to feel like I wasn't a freak of nature, or that I hadn't just missed the pick-up date for the human owner's manual on how to live life. The chain that bound me to perceived terminal uniqueness was broken. (I still revisit the idea of uniqueness from time to time, and can get sucked into romancing the dark underground of my youth, but I don't stay there too long and it doesn't take over anymore.) Step Two brought hope to my life. It was in the group that I felt a connection to a Power Greater than myself, that the fellowship was bigger than me. I may need to be restored to sanity, but I don't have to do it by myself. I wrote this last sentence in the present tense because restoration is an ongoing process and we don't actually graduate with a certificate of sanity.

Modern day spiritualists have been known to reject the principle of hope by teaching that the wanting or striving for hope in itself implies a statement of lack. The idea is that if we're hoping for something, we are affirming we don't have it, and we don't want to promote or confirm lack on an energetic level, so let's take hope out of the equation. I get the basic premise, but I wholeheartedly feel that hope is an essential principle for recovery. For those that are already living in lack, or are already totally hopeless, hope is a stepping stone to coming to believe. That being said, you can approach your search for hope in a positive way.

The hope talked about in Step Two is not akin to a wish, like when you were a kid hoping for a shiny, new bike or Barbie Dream House, complete with elevator, for your birthday. It is a hope that moves in and takes residence in the body, easing and alleviating doubt. Hope may creep in slowly, and then grow deeply with experience in recovery. Step Two asks us to stay in the moment, do what is in front of us right now, as we build belief in the possibility of long-term recovery.

This step does not require a belief in God, but for some people this comes naturally. Our beliefs and spiritual practices vary from the religiously devout to the atheist. Be assured, all are welcome and no specific belief or religion is required. All are encouraged to experiment with what works for them and eliminate what doesn't. What's really important is simply being open and willing to seek connection. Referring back to Chapter 3, simply being open and willing is essentially true for yoga as well. You have been given the power of choice in Step One and you get to use it again in Step Two.

The connection to the group can be a great way to begin the journey into believing it can work for you, too. There is power in the group, a connection, communion, and acceptance that is palpable. We gain hope, and little by little we begin to believe the program can work for us because we see it working for others. Our belief grows until one day we're living it and helping others, too. Hope is the principle that ushers in belief, an authentic belief that goes beyond the intellect.

One of my favorite lines from the AA Big Book is *"What an order, I can't go through with it."* It makes me smile now, because we all have some degree of resistance and rebellion when we first get to the program, and maybe we maintain it for years to come, but ultimately the work is very much accessible because we only have to do it for today. Just one measly day, that's all. We only have to abstain and be present for today. Tomorrow is another story that has not yet arrived.

I remember being hit hard with cravings to use when I had about 18 months clean and sober. It was a smoggy day in Los Angeles, gray on the outside like I felt on the inside, and I wanted to use drugs. I was on the freeway wallowing in my own sorrowful, gray mood, and thought I could easily take an exit coming up to get to the connection. I was so up in my head, not liking the way I was feeling, and wanting escape. In all of my years of recovery I have never been so tempted to return to the insanity. I went back and forth with myself, and made the decision that if I still felt like this the following day I would go get loaded. Something immediately clicked and I started laughing out loud. After 18 months of hearing just for today, or one day at a time, it finally made sense and that's exactly what I was doing, applying it to my real-life situation. I recall telling myself something along the lines of, *"You idiot, that's how the program works, I just don't use today!"* I continued to laugh along my drive, the urge to use was lifted, and I was truly granted insight into the simplicity of the 12 Step program. 'Just for today' came to life.

For a frame of reference, we had no cell phones back then, and only the big shots had beepers. The pager, sadly, was not my path. Today it is easier to reach out to someone anytime, as you don't need to be sitting at a home phone or have a quarter for the payphone. I'm laughing to myself now because some of you have never had to use a payphone in your life. Before, during, or after an experience such as I described above, it is always a good idea to check in with a sponsor or friends. It's other people who have paved the way for us to walk our path, and support us in our growth. I'm a big believer that God works through people.

We cannot afford to fool ourselves into thinking that we can change our external world without doing the internal work. Recovery is an inside job. We must change the inside so that it reflects on the outside.

Testimonial:

"Although I am a "newbie" to the practice of yoga, I have been a member of 12 step recovery programs for the majority of my life. Like recovery, yoga, for me, is a light in the darkness. It is an opportunity to freely heal and be friends with my soul again. Kundalini yoga is spiritually grounding to me in a profound way. When we practice meditating together, I feel connected to myself, my fellow human beings, and the Creator. There is an indescribable feeling of well-being that comes from being fully in the present moment. I experience an amazing energy of acceptance and love as well as the presence of community." - Ann M.

Bonus:

Yogurt Detox Bath Recipe

This recipe is for external use only. Ingestion is not recommended.
Ingredients:
½ Gallon of natural, plain yogurt
Juice of one Lemon
Dab of honey

Directions:

Let the yogurt sit out of the refrigerator overnight or all day, and then mix the ingredients together. Sit in an empty bathtub and rub the body with the mixture. Massage the body briskly with the yogurt mixture. Continue to scoop up and rub in for 20 minutes. Cover all parts of the body, including the hair. After about 20 minutes take a warm shower and wash as normal. Your body literally drinks in the yogurt. This is very moisturizing. If the yogurt turns gray, don't worry, you're just eliminating toxins.

This recipe was shared with me years ago by a fellow yoga teacher and friend.

Yoga Recommendation:

Kirtan Kriya is a powerful meditation for mental cleansing and clearing. It is recommended for Step Two for its positive affect on the mind. The movement and mantra provide the second chakra focus and flow, and an overall connection with something bigger than the self.

Emotional Balance & Repair of Damage Due to Cocaine (Drug) Use with Kirtan Kriya Yoga Meditation

A. In meditation pose, with a straight spine, do Breath of Fire for 31 minutes. (You may build up to 31 minutes by starting with 3 to 5 minutes and adding time slowly.)

B. Kirtan Kriya for 31 minutes. Meditate at the Brow Point, chanting the 5 primal sounds of the Panj Shabad. (You may begin with 12 minutes, cutting the times proportionately.)

Sa – Infinity, cosmos, beginning
Ta – life, existence
Na - death
Ma – rebirth

Hands on knees, elbows straight, on "Sa" touch the Jupiter (index) finger to the thumb. On "Ta" touch the Saturn (middle) finger to the thumb. On "Na" touch the thumb and the Sun (ring) finger, and on "Ma" touch the Mercury (pinky) finger and thumb. Repeat and continue.

For the first 5 minutes, chant in a normal voice (language of the human), for the next 5 minutes, whisper (language of lovers), and for the next 10 minutes chant silently (divine language). For the next 5 minutes come back to the whispered chanting, and for the last 5 minutes return to the normal voice. (These are the 3 languages of consciousness.) Meditate on the 4 primal sounds in a "L" shape. Let each "Sa Ta Na Ma" enter through the crown chakra, or top of the head, and project it out to infinity through the brow point, or 3rd eye.

Comments:

These are the most effective tools we can apply. The results are 100% effective. Kirtan Kriya is the most important meditation in Kundalini Yoga. If you could do only one, this is it! It does everything for you in the proper order! It is powerful for emotional balance. If you can't 'get it together," do this meditation for 31 minutes and be totally balanced. Over a period of time, this meditation can be your best friend.

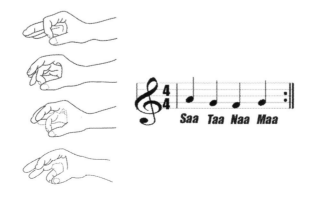

10

Step Three

"We made a decision to turn our will and our lives over the care of God as we understood Him."

"Surrendering is the opposite of giving up, it is giving over." -Gabrielle Bernstein (2016)

The key word for Step Three is decision. The key concepts are letting go and turning it over. We make a decision to turn our will over, we surrender our way, and ask for direction and help, and then we spend years to come doing it over and over again. Not to sound discouraging, we may need only make one big decision and then do the footwork necessary to support our decision. Remember, it's simply a decision to step into faith. The direction to make this decision in Step Three reminds us first and foremost that we are not in control and we need continued and greater help if we are to maintain our recovery. Making a decision to turn it over and leaving the results to God sounds fine and dandy, but how do we take the action to initiate this type of letting go followed by a reliance on faith and trust?

This step takes us from a Power Greater than ourselves in Step Two, to a God of our understanding. It is asking you to dig deeper and make a bigger commitment. But don't worry, you still have the power of choice. You get to decide about the God of your understanding, not your sponsor, your friends, your family, or recovery literature. You get to decide! It's also ok if you are undecided at this point, all that is needed is an openness to the idea that there could be a God or Higher Power with whom at some point you may wish to build a relationship. Continue using the fellowship, the group, the steps, etc., as your connection to something greater than yourself as long as needed. Yogic principles may help in the process, as they teach that we are an embodiment of the Divine, and we are taught to see ourselves as an expression of the Divine. This does not mean we're running things, but rather we already have all we need, and we may look for connection within rather than without.

For those who have religion and a tradition that resonates for them, by all means return to the comforting roots of churches, temples, mosques, and/or ashrams. The Basic Text of Narcotics Anonymous suggests that you choose a God that is a loving force, but that is really the only guideline given in regard to a Higher Power.

For the non-believer or atheist, do not fret; I know from personal experience that you can still work this step. On my very first night in residential treatment, as I crawled into the bottom bunk, one of my roommates reminded all of us in the room to pray before going to sleep. Internally I was like, *"No way, I did not come here to find God."* I was exhausted and just wanted to bundle up in a warm bed. My very first prayer in recovery came shortly after this first evening, and went something along the lines of *"Hey God, it's me, you know I don't believe, but I'm willing to be open. I need help."* I would not admit to this prayer and the experience for some months to come. We'll revisit this story in Step Twelve. The honest action we are willing to take in Step Two builds and affirms the faith and trust needed for Step Three.

Now, what exactly do we need to let go of? Well, pretty much everything, just like what we need to change is everything. This letting go is more about getting out of our own way, not obsessing on details, and learning that we can take action but stay out of the results. Trying to control and manage our own lives has not worked, so we are asked to try another way. Many times, this may play out as not making decisions on our own, and instead asking for input from within our trusted recovery community. From our early days in recovery my husband has been adamant that Step Three is about making new and different choices. It's adjacent to taking contrary action. For example, if my head says do this, I'll talk to someone and probably end up doing the opposite. Once we've made a decision, whether we decide to have spinach salad for dinner or decide to look for a new job, we are then invited to stay out of the driver's seat. We are advised to not be attached to the results as we make plans and take action.

The results are not our business. How can we in our limited, and possibly dysfunctional thinking, assume that we know what is in our best interest. We may be granted much more than we had even dared hope to achieve. A regular practice of yoga and meditation take us beyond superficial thinking to the awakening of intuition. With developed intuition comes the guidance to make better choices. In the meantime, we are asked to have faith and trust in a Higher Power, get out of our own way, and be open to the delivery.

Getting out of our own way is not always easy because as human beings we long for security and safety, which in turn drives our desire to control our inner and outer environments. Life does not come with any guarantees. Grasping at security and safety keeps us stuck in the familiar and is futile because both are an illusion. Chasing security actually creates insecurity. Again, we are faced with the invitation to trust in the divine flow of life, and yoga is a wonderful practice to embody an allowing of trust while maintaining inner peace.

I already mentioned that turning it over is about stepping into faith, but we also need to do the footwork. Having faith without footwork is a dead-end road. For example, say you need to find a new apartment and you've been praying for it to come to fruition. That's great, but are you actually looking for a new place to live? Are you actively seeking apartments online, filling out applications, talking to friends, or asking around? Or are you praying, then parking yourself on the couch eating potato chips and binging Netflix while waiting for the Universe to deliver your new apartment? An effective Step Three calls for both action and faith in the outcome.

Not only are we able to turn the results of our own lives over to the care of a Power Greater than ourselves, but we can turn others over, too. I have had to apply this to my relationship with my kids throughout the years. It is not my business to plan, execute, and manage their lives just because I love and worry about them. Even with love and the best of intentions, it's not my job to run their lives. I got called out on this by my sponsor a few years back when she asked me if I had faith that God has a plan for me and if I believe my needs would be met. When I answered yes, she questioned why I didn't believe that to be true for my children as well. I think I was stunned into silence. Not only do we turn over our will, but we turn over our will for others as well. We don't' get to decide what is best for others.

This action step of faith may actually feel like a tug of war as we turn it over, take it back, turn it over, take it back, and finally let it go until we come up with a better idea and take it back again, exhaust all efforts, and in our despair turn it over and finally release the results. Step Three cultivates the habit of letting go. An internal tug of war may manifest in many different areas of life, but we have the choice to let go of the rope at any time.

It's time to interject a bit of helpful information here and state that spirit is not emotion, but rather beyond our emotions. Feelings are messages that we receive from the environment in order to help us decipher and move through life, but feelings are not spirit and they are not our true identity. They give us a ton of information and it's up to us to determine what next action may or may not be useful in any given situation. Yoga asks us to channel emotion into devotion, and develop reverence for all. This is a nice companion for Step Three. Listen to your feelings, but don't mistake them for your spirit.

Devotion is beyond the realm of thought. Your thoughts are not who you really are, and they may not accurately represent your true belief system. In the yogic philosophy it is said that we have more than 1,000 thoughts per wink of the eye and we are largely unaware of the vast majority. We occasionally hit on one that we attach to, which gives it energy to grow. Be aware of old, self-defeating, repetitive thoughts and self-talk, and shift toward being conscious of your thoughts and projections. Step Three can help with making this shift because we move beyond the individual self as the center of the world. Step Two suggests that we will need others on our journey, and now Step Three includes a Higher

Divine Power, thus duplicating the flow of individual, group, and universal consciousness as a natural path to faith, as is found in the yogic path.

Faith in motion is learning to live with trust through times of uncertainty, and through personal experience, a development of an inner knowing that all is well. No matter what life delivers, it is all going to be okay. Make a decision, and let it go. There are no guarantees. Apprehension may abound and linger. Do it anyway.

It is a good idea to at least occasionally make this decision out loud, and remember to give thanks. Verbally affirm the decision to turn your will and your life over to the care of a power greater than yourself, and be open to expansion.

Testimonial:

"I have been in a 12 Step recovery program for 30 years. This practice is such a natural addition to my program. At the core of my recovery, the realm of the spirit is broad, roomy, and all inclusive, and Kundalini yoga is a perfect match for me and my spirituality. And, I feel GREAT!" - Lonnie M.

Bonus:

Keep it Simple Activity

Make a list of five thoughts, attitudes, and/or behaviors you can cultivate on a regular basis to help you remember to keep it simple. I have included this activity in step three because many people struggle with intellectualizing the concept of a Higher Power, as well as the process of letting go, before dropping into pure experience.

If there's a harder way of doing something, mankind will surely figure it out; however, it is not necessary when working the steps. A little analogy plugged in here may be a helpful reminder to keep you on track. When going into space, the United States spent many man hours and millions of dollars to create a pen that would write in zero gravity, whereas the Russians used a pencil. Are you trying to reinvent the pen, or are you using a pencil?

Yoga Recommendation:

The third chakra is the navel chakra, the fire element, the seat of personal power and physical health. Both the third chakra and the Third Step are about the integration of information and finding a place within community where the focus is on the greater good. This *kriya* is chosen in order to build navel point power, and to move from an attitude of *me* to embracing the concept of *we*.

Kriya to Develop Navel Intelligence

This kriya is for strengthening the navel point. Begin with one minute of each exercise and slowly work up to the stated time as you develop your ability to do the exercise correctly.

1. Sit on your heels, rooting through your sit bones. Interlock your fingers in Venus Lock behind your neck. Spread your shoulder blades apart as you point your elbows out to the sides. Lift your chest up into Neck Lock and begin Breath of Fire. 2 minutes.

2. Lie on your stomach, rooting through your navel point into the floor. Bend your knees. Reach back, grab your ankles, and press them toward your buttocks. Keep your chest on the ground. Breathe normally. Hold the position for 2 minutes.

3. Stretch Pose. Lie on your back, rooting through the small of your back so that it presses into the floor. Raise your head and heels six inches off the floor. Point the hands toward your toes and begin Breath of Fire. 2 minutes. Keep yourself rooted so that the small of your back is pressed against the floor. If your back lifts off the floor, keep your breath going, but come down, re-establish your root line, and come back up into the posture. To do Stretch Pose correctly, you'll find that your will have to be in Neck Lock. The chest must be lifted to support the head. If you collapse your chest to get your head off the ground, it pressures your lower back to sway up.

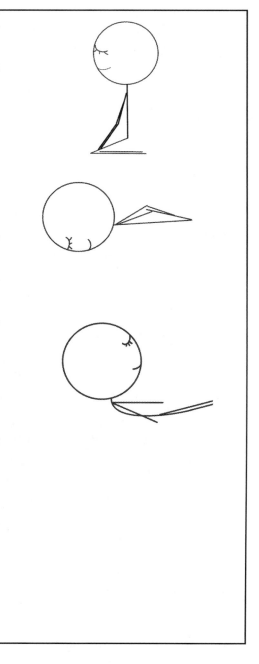

4. Lie on your back. Bring your left knee to your chest as you extend your right leg out straight, parallel to the ground. Then bring your right knee to your chest as you extend your left leg out straight. Continue alternately moving the legs in a piston-like motion. Keep your navel engaged so that your lower back stays rooted to the floor. Breathe deeply. 2 minutes.

5. Lie on your back, keep your lower back rooted to the floor. Inhale and lift both legs up to ninety degrees. Exhale and keep the root line as you lower your legs. Keep your legs together with your toes pointed. Continue raising and lowering both legs with powerful breathing for 2 minutes. On the inhale up, feel as if the breath is lifting your legs. On the exhale down use the navel to brake against gravity.

6. King Cobra. Lie on your stomach, with your hands under your shoulders. Root through your abdomen into the floor and raise your chest. Slowly arch up into Cobra Pose as far as you can without compressing your lower back. Once you are up in the arch, bend your knees and raise your feet up toward your head. Hold 2 minutes. (When your internal framework is strong enough to protect your neck from compression, you can release your head backward to touch your feet.)

Modify by remaining in Cobra Pose, lifting into an arch only as far as is comfortable for the spine.

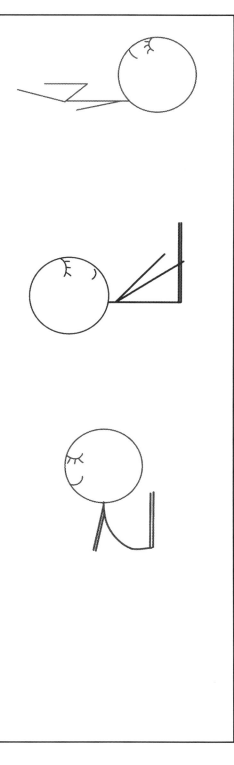

7. Lie on your back, bringing your knees to your chest to counter-balance the last position. Hold briefly and then roll forward and backward on your spine. Continue for 2 minutes.

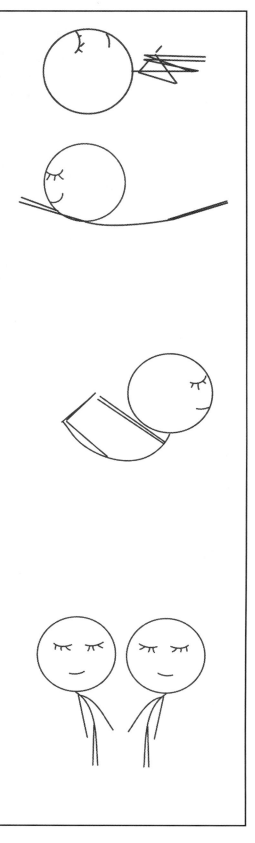

8. Lie on your stomach with your arms extended in front of you, palms together. Create a root line through your abdomen into the floor and raise your arms and legs off the ground. Hold this position with Breath of Fire for 2 minutes. Ideally you should feel you lower back elongating, as if someone is pulling your feet in one direction while someone else pulls your arms in the opposite direction.

9. Bow Pose. Lie on your stomach, once again rooting through your lower abdomen. Reach back and grasp your ankles. Use your legs to pull against your arms and raise yourself up into Bow Pose. Hold the position with Breath of Fire for 2 minutes.

   Modify by raising up in the direction of Bow Pose, without actually holding the ankles, by leaving the elbows and palms on the floor, or by using a yoga strap to reach and hold around the ankles.

10. Stand up in Mountain Pose. (Stand with your feet together, with both Root Lock and Neck Lock applied.) Stretch the arms out to the sides, parallel to the ground with the palms facing down. Without twisting your torso, inhale and bend to the left, exhale and bend to the right. Rhythmically stretch your ribs open, bending left and right. Maintain your grip on the root line to maximize the stretch along the side of the rib cage. 2 minutes.

11. Still standing, spread your feet one and one half to two feet apart. Twist your torso to the left, swinging the left arm out to the side, parallel to the floor with the palm facing forward. At the same time, bring your right palm to the center of your chest. Then quickly change arms as your twist to the other side. Continue twisting from side to side while alternating the arms positions. Inhale as your left arms swings outward and you twist left, exhale as your right arm swings outward and your twist right. Continue for 2 minutes. Move from the navel.

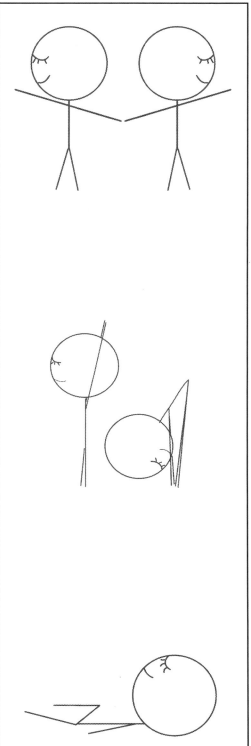

12. Stand with the feet hip-width apart. Raise your arms over your head with the heels of your palms pressing upward. Root through your feet and draw your kneecaps up. Inhale in this position, lifting your chest and arching slightly backward. (Press your shoulder blades down to keep your chest lifted and protect your backward arch.) Exhale and bend forward at the navel point, bringing your hands to the floor. Inhale and root your feet into the floor, using the big muscle of your legs to push yourself upright. Continue bending forward and rising up. 2 minutes. If you cannot touch the floor when bending forward, go only as far as your range of motion allows.

13. Lie on your back and repeat exercise #4, remembering to root through the lower back, keeping contact with the floor. 2 minutes.

14. Lie on your back. Inhale and keep your lower back pressed against the floor as your raise your left leg up to ninety degrees. Exhale as you lower the leg, keeping the lower back pressed against the floor. Inhale and raise your right leg up to ninety degrees. Exhale as your lower it. Continue alternate leg lifts. Breathe deeply and fully. Continue for 2 minutes.

15. Come in to the position for Sat Kriya. (Described in Chapter 8.) Squeeze your navel on "Sat" and relax the navel on "Naam." Do not neglect the relaxation on "Naam." Allow your navel point to release before you engage it again. Roll your armpits toward each other to keep your arms hugging your ears. Continue for 2 minutes. Then inhale deeply, hold the breath, apply the Mula bandh (Root Lock). Hold for a long as you comfortably can. Exhale and relax on your back for 2 minutes.

16. Sit straight with your legs extended out in front of you. Throughout this exercise, keep a strong Neck Lock and Root Lock to maintain the integrity of the heart center. Do not allow your chest to collapse. Lean back to sixty degrees and raise your legs up to sixty degrees. Extend your arms parallel to the ground with the palms facing down. Hold this position with Breath of Fire. 2 minutes. Modified version is pictured.

If the lower back requires additional support, you can bend the knees slightly. The bigger the bend, the more pressure released from the lower back.

17. Lie down on your back and totally relax.

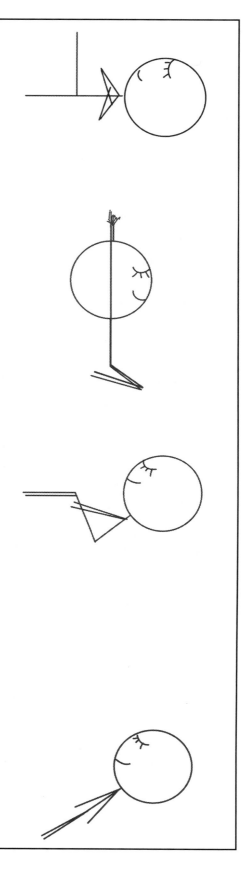

11

Step Four

"We made a searching and fearless moral inventory of ourselves."

"The things that upset you are an entry point into understanding yourself and healing the wounds that are at the source of your reactions." -GuruMeher Khalsa (2021)

Step Four gives direction for a searching and fearless moral inventory, which sounds daunting, but is actually pretty straightforward. We take inventory to see what we're working with, not to beat ourselves up or try to impress our sponsor with what a badass we are, but to take stock of ourselves in a truthful way. We may begin to do this by taking a look at our resentments because they are clues to any dis-ease we're holding on to from the past. In Step Four it is time to address the emotions that have been driving our destructive behavior. What most of us have not learned, and by "us" I'm not referring to addicts only, but humanity in general, is that our emotions serve to give us information and guidance. Feelings literally give us input, and they do not have to be labeled as good or bad. When children aren't taught to talk about and how to handle their big and little feelings, or aren't allowed to have feelings at all, this can transpose as trauma response behavior in adulthood. This step is an opportunity to dig deep, take a look at unresolved feelings and the repercussions of hanging on to them, whether suppressed or overtly expressed, so we may continue to find balance and heal.

Step working guides and literature differ within each 12 Step program, but one common theme is writing about resentments. Resentments are a sneaky, silent killer, allowing one to justify thought and deed and hold on to blame. As long as we stay in a cycle of anger, we will find no freedom. It is only through taking responsibility that we are granted freedom. I may have mentioned this in Step One, and it is also true here in the Fourth Step. Step Four provides an opportunity to blame, express anger, and point fingers. That's not all. Step Four takes us full circle so we fully look at our part and then finally urges us to let go of long held patterns of pain. It is an effective tool for giving up a running list of grudges.

What do you mean, running list of grudges? You know, that invisible clipboard hanging off your belt where you may keep a tally of all trespasses, real or perceived, that have offended the oh so delicate self. The clipboard goes everywhere to aid in keeping score. A check mark may easily be added to the running list, and new names can be added at any time. The list may be one-sided, but it is all-inclusive. The list of grudges functions as a shield to keep distance between self and others and to maintain an air of self-righteousness. I was conspicuous in the maintaining of my personal list. If this does not sound familiar, please look again before completely releasing the possibility that you're holding grudges.

Courage is the principle for Step Four and we draw on it to take honesty to the next level for the purpose of letting go of resentments and being accountable for ourselves in all areas of life. The courage required for a complete self-assessment is utilized in order to release blame, heal past traumas, and ultimately gain freedom from our personal secrets. You know, the stuff we swore we'd take to the grave, the stuff we're too ashamed to share with anyone else, the stuff we don't even want to think about ourselves. Step Four is the work done between ourselves and a Higher Power. Let go of the following Step Five while doing this work and stay in today.

A few years back I was having a conversation with a friend and yoga student, actually more of an informal interview for her dissertation. She was questioning the fear and resistance people have to being totally honest and living in truth as it relates to a yogic lifestyle, both in the past and modern-day life. The only answer that came to me was a Jack Nicholson line from *A Few Good Men, "YOU CAN'T HANDLE THE TRUTH!"* Most of us want to be assured of a comfortable truth that easily fits into our view of life, but this is not reality. This step is a really big deal, but guess what, you can handle it, and you don't have to do it alone.

Early on in recovery a mentor suggested to me that I had the concept of "cash register honesty," but lacked courage to take a good look at myself. She explained that cash register honesty is the ability to tell the cashier they gave you $20 in change when you were only owed $10, and then you give the money back. Yes, that's being honest, but it's only on a superficial level. My mentor then went on to state I needed to take more than a quick peek inside, that I needed to really spend some time looking within. She then gave a physical demonstration that has always stayed with me. She pulled her shirt collar out and took a brief glance inside then let the collar lie flat again with quick sigh of relief, signifying that all is well, nothing going on here, *phew* that's over. She explained that a quick glance was the current extent of my willingness. She then pulled her shirt collar out, tilted her head down, and took a nice long look inside, moving her eyes around to see all, and then told me that's what I needed to do in order to recover. I was scared of what would happen if I actually tackled the arduous task of finding out who I really am, and discovered I didn't like her.

Although courage is the principle behind this step, fear can be a motivating factor. I listened to people in meetings, both those who stayed, and those who returned after relapsing, and tried to figure out how it all worked. When it was time to work Step Four and write my personal inventory, all I knew was that I didn't want to feel the way I felt walking in the door my first day clean, and I did not want to return to a lifestyle of active addiction and its accompanying sidekicks, desperation and degradation. Sometimes what we don't want motivates us to work toward what we do want. Fear of what would happen if I didn't work this step gave me courage to walk through it and to do my best to be honest.

As a result, a couple of things happened. First, I realized that I am accountable for my own life, that yes, there were past traumas to heal, but trying to blame others for my unhappiness was both senseless and ridiculous. When there's one finger pointing out, there are four pointing back at me. In yoga this is described in a way that all people we encounter, and all people we have relationships with, simply offer us a mirror; they reflect ourselves back to us. So, we are asked to be honest and write everything, as our secrets will only keep us sick and stuck. In working this step, my second realization was that as humans we all experience similar feelings and our similarities outweigh our differences.

In taking responsibility I had to let my parents off the hook. I'll share this story because it was so clear to me that my dissatisfaction was about me, not the attitudes and behavior of those around me. Yes, I had childhood wounds to heal, and this is not about diminishing any painful circumstances or fragile feelings, but rather learning how not to drag them with me into every current and future relationship. As I began to write about resentments, I felt completely justified in my anger. However, as I continued to write I began to see patterns that revealed no matter what action my parents took or did not take, I was not going to be satisfied. For example, in my day in and day out trials and tribulations, if they said nothing to me, I could translate that as that as they don't care or I don't matter. If they actually did address something about me or my behavior then I would be mad, and translate their concern as butting in, meddling, disapproval, etc. It was truly a case of damned if you do, damned if you don't, originating from the way I felt about myself. This pattern played out in all of my relationships based on my own unexpressed feelings and expectations. Once I saw my part, I was able to drop some of my angry armor. I'm over-simplifying here to make my point, but I honestly had no insight into this revelation before I did the actual work of writing a Fourth Step.

The writing of a Fourth Step may not be a one-and-done deal. As progress is made in recovery more is revealed and there may be times that require revisiting Step Four for additional exposure, sharing, and healing. I was a couple of years, okay decades, into recovery when I was really ready, willing and cognizant of the fact that I needed to go back to my childhood for further forgiveness through writing a very specific Fourth Step. I was able to heal deep sadness and shame. This does not mean that the first attempt at a Fourth Step was not successful; it simply means we deal with the layers as they come up and we address what is most pressing first. The most pressing issues are usually on the surface. We clean up the surface and then move deeper into the layers, like unpeeling an onion. For example, first we may have to work on guilt and then later shame. Guilt is an emotion we carry and shame is an identity we build. Shame has a firmly embedded grasp because it's about who we are, not only how we feel about what we have done. We begin with what's present and take one step at a time, write one word at a time, take deep breaths one at a time, and exercise the body one day at a time.

The peeling of the onion may at times feel redundant. What I mean by this is that reoccurring themes or problems in our lives will surface in different ways until we learn the intended lesson or do the necessary healing. Running away to escape the self is no longer a viable option. There is a saying in yoga, *"Keep up and you will be kept up."*

As we explore our inner, emotional landscape we may come to realize that our perception of events is ours alone. Another gift of Step Four is that it allows us to let go of holding others accountable for our perception. Life events don't have to be saved up for a future inventory; issues may be addressed as they arise. Each time we find ourselves revisiting old, familiar feelings of regret or sadness, we have the tools to release internalized feelings from the past so that they don't spoil today.

As humans, we spend a great deal of our time ruminating over the past or projecting into the future. Recovery from addiction happens right now in the present moment. The practice of yoga, whether it be breath, meditation, or posture, supports this step because its very nature is to bring the practitioner into current time and space, or the present moment. When we have one foot in yesterday and one foot in tomorrow, we miss today. We can become so comfortable in the familiar stories we have carried with us through life that our story begins to feel concrete and real. The attachment to these stories and fear of the unknown keeps us trapped and repeating the same cycles over and over. Yoga describes this attachment as *maya*, or the illusion of reality. One of the secrets to happiness is to step outside of our personal box of comfort, even if we're afraid, and Step Four definitely fits the bill of stepping beyond what is comfortable.

Addiction is characterized by complete self-centeredness. There is a program saying that sums it up well. *"I may not be much, but I'm all I think about."* Each person will deal with different issues in the Fourth Step based on their own experiences and perceptions of life. The commonality lies in the feelings behind the issues, whether they be anger, insecurity, fear, low self-esteem, rejection, isolation, shame, guilt, etc. Step Four takes us both into, and out of, the self in order to gain clarity and awareness, which helps us heal and make better choices in the future. The pain cracks our outer protective shell, and then gives a push to stretch beyond the confines of a self-imposed prison. Through this cracking, or coming apart, we blossom. We can stop keeping score and get rid of the grudge list. The cracking of the shell also reveals our personal strengths. Empowerment lies in personally working through the tough outer shell, not by being crushed from outside forces. The process of finding out and owning who we are can foster greater love and acceptance of self and others.

Yogic philosophy, through the 8 limbs, gives us a broader view of our purpose, and softens self-assessment through emphasizing appraisal without judgement. The teachings indicate that we are given this particular life path, and all the people we encounter on this path, to learn needed soul lessons and to play our part in helping others learn their lessons. From this perspective, we see that all of our life experiences are necessary for us to become who we really are, and for the greater growth of our soul body. This is the perfect opportunity to decrease our victim mentality. It is your choice to be the victim or the victor. It could be that something you went through and healed in yourself is going to give you the chance to help someone else through the same healing process. We are afforded healing from physical, emotional and sexual abuse, lying, cheating, dishonesty, poor self-worth, harm both endured and inflicted, guilt, shame, insecurity, resentment, abandonment, neglect, illness, loss and grief, and the trauma that accumulated from such experiences. We are welcomed to edit and re-write our own story from here on out. All of the combined life experiences thus far have led you to this moment in time, to who you are today. Yoga and recovery ask you to be who you are, honestly and completely.

Testimonial:

"A lot of people struggle with the 4th Step of AA or any other 12-Step program. Some of us were in denial about things that happened to us and things we did because of our drinking and drugs. To drag it all up and tell it to another person (5th Step) is very painful. But it is important to come to terms with the past – and a great relief to share it and stop carrying it around inside of us like a stone of guilt and shame. I started doing Kundalini Yoga when I had six years of sobriety, and it has been a wonderful companion in my AA journey for 22 years ... and counting. The teachings are the same. Accept yourself, open your heart to a higher level of consciousness and wisdom, and learn to live in the world." - Adesh Kaur

Bonus:

Guided Meditation

I Am in the Right Place

"Everything I need comes to me in the perfect time-space sequence. Just as all the stars and planets are in their perfect orbit and in Divine right order, so am I. I may not understand everything that is going on with my limited human mind; however, I know that on the cosmic level, I must be in the right place, at the right time, doing the right thing. Positive thoughts are what I choose to think. This present experience is a stepping-stone to a new awareness and greater glory." -Lousie L. Hay, Inner Wisdom (2000)

Yoga Recommendation:

A *kriya* for eliminating anger has been chosen for Step Four in order to release feelings of grief, resentment, and betrayal held within the body. These are the feelings addressed at the core of this step, and this physical practice helps to heal the heart center, or fourth chakra, by releasing suppressed anger. Compassion and forgiveness are fostered as anger lessens.

Take a few moments to explore your why. Make a list of what motivates you on a personal level:

Kriya to Relieve Inner Anger

Inner anger blocks your relationships with others because it blocks your relationship with yourself. This powerful set works to effectively release and transform inner anger.

1. Sleep Pose. Lie down on your back in a relaxed posture with your arms at your side, palms up, and your legs slightly apart. Close the eyes and pretend to snore. Continue for 1 ½ minutes.

2. Leg Hold #1. Still lying on the back, keep your legs straight and raise both legs 6 inches above the ground and hold. Breathe normally for 2 minutes. This exercise balances anger. It applies pressure to the navel to balance the entire system.

3. Leg Hold #2. Still lying on the back with the legs 6 inches above the ground, stretch the tongue out and begin Breath of Fire through the mouth for 1 ½ minutes.

4. Beat the Ground. Still lying on the back, lift the legs perpendicular to the floor, resting the arms on the ground by the sides, palms down. Begin to beat the ground with all the anger you can achieve. Beat hard and fast, using the entire length of the arms. Continue for 2 ½ minutes.

5. Knees to Chest. Bring the knees to the chest and wrap the arms around them. Stretch the tongue out. Inhale through the open mouth and exhale through the nose. Continue for 1 to 2 minutes.

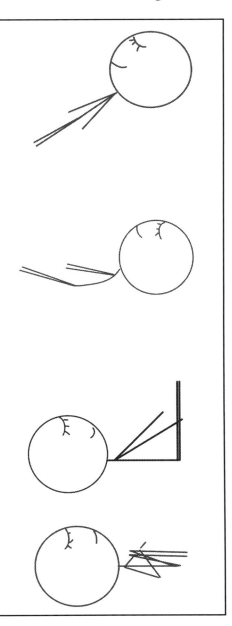

6. Celibate Pose Bends. From a position of sitting on your heels, move your heels out to the sides so that your buttocks are resting on the floor. Spread your knees as far apart as possible. Cross the arms over the chest and press them hard against your rib cage. Bend forward and touch the forehead to the floor as if you are bowing. Exhale as your go down, inhale up. Go for 2 ½ minutes at a pace of approximately one bow every 2 seconds. Then for 30 seconds speed up and move as fast as you can. Modify by staying in Rock or Easy Pose.

7. Self-Massage. Sit with the legs straight out in front of you. Begin to beat all parts of your body with open palms. Move quickly for 2 minutes.

8. Hang Loose. Stand up. Bend forward, keeping your back parallel to the ground, and let your arms and hands hang loose. If available, sing along with a recording of Guru Ram Das Chant as your hang. Remain in this posture for 1 to 3 minutes.

9. Cobra Pose. Lie on the stomach with the palms flat on the floor under the shoulders. The heels are together, and the tops of the feet are on the floor. Inhale into Cobra Pose, stretching the spine, vertebra by vertebra, from the neck to the base of the spine as far as possible. The arms may be slightly bent at the elbow to ensure that the shoulders are not tensed. Make sure to stretch the head out of the neck, and relax the shoulders downward. Exhale. Continue to sing with the Guru Ram Das Chant, if possible, while in Cobra for 1 minute. Then, still in Cobra and singing, begin to circle the head around on the neck both ways for a total of 30 seconds. Still in Cobra Pose, begin kicking the ground with alternate feet. Continue for 30 seconds.

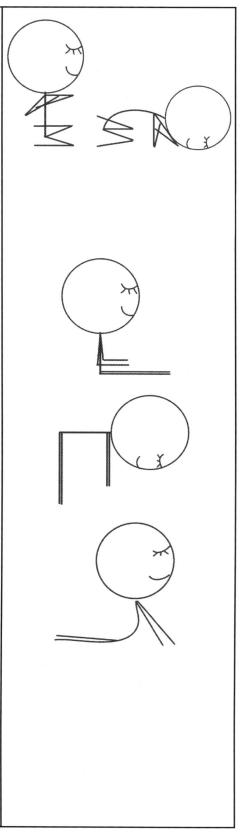

10. Sat Kriya in Easy Pose for 1 minute. Stretch the arms up with the elbows hugging the sides of the head. Interlock all the fingers except the index fingers of each hand, which are pointing straight up. Begin to say the sound "Sat" as you pull the navel up and in toward the spine. As you say "Nam," relax the belly area. Chant emphatically in a constant rhythm about 8 times per 10 seconds. Then, inhale and squeeze the muscles tightly from the buttocks all the way up the back, past the shoulders. Mentally allow the energy to flow through the head and out the top of the skull. Exhale and relax. This exercise circulates the kundalini energy and integrates the energy released from the lower three chakras into the entire system, so that the total effects of these exercises are stable and long lasting.

11. Lie down on the back for deep relaxation for at least 5 minutes.

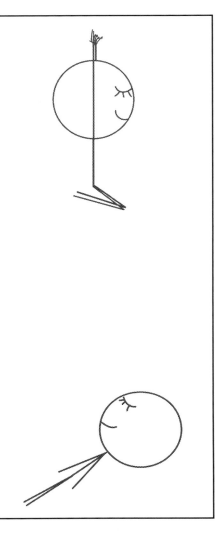

12

Step Five

"We admitted to God, to ourselves, and to another human being the exact nature of our wrongs."

"Judgement is the reverberation of a soul experiencing the unconscious state of separation." - The Poetry of Michael

Now that the work of writing a moral inventory is done, we are asked to share it with another trusted human being, usually a sponsor. Family members, best friends, and buddies from our days of drinking and using are not appropriate choices for this step. You are asked to take a leap of faith in following through with Step Five. It may be helpful to focus on trusting the process of recovery, even if you don't yet trust yourself. This is one reason it is important to have a sponsor, a person experienced working steps in the program.

The principle of Step Five is integrity. Your integrity and the integrity of the person with whom you choose to share are combined for this experience of unveiling and letting go. Shady people and hidden agendas are not conducive to a positive Fifth Step outcome. Employ the heart, not the head, when making the decision on who will receive and honor the responsibility of listening to your Fifth Step. The heart center holds the neutral mind and is your best source of guidance.

When our moral inventory is heard and received without judgment, but with understanding, we are disarmed. When secrets are exposed and feelings are validated, we create space for healing. A lifetime of self-armoring can begin to break apart and fall away to reveal the true self when we take the risk and open up to another human being. Imagine the protective armor to be like tiles on the roof of a house, overlapping to provide full coverage, and secured in place by the builder. Now picture a strong wind blowing through the house causing the house to creak and move, a few tiles to crack, lift, and maybe even fall to the ground. Liken this image to taking a deep breath of relief after sharing Step Five where the secrets have been revealed. Visualize a deep inhale, a breath so full that the rib cage is able to expand causing pieces of personal armor, like the tiles of the roof, to loosen and wiggle, and then with the exhale see the armor begin to break and fall off, dropping to the ground. Losing the protective armor, or letting the wall of defenses down, does not happen overnight or in one fell swoop, rather it is an ongoing process through recovery. Step Five is a big step toward shedding the suit of armor.

Valid concerns with the ramifications of sharing all wrong-doings with another person may be a very real issue, which is worth careful consideration. Each individual will have to assess whether sharing certain aspects of their lives will bring them harm, such as sharing openly actions that may lead to incarceration. I actually know recovering people who turned themselves in to serve a short sentence to clean up the wreckage of their past, but this is not required. My point is that sharing your Fifth Step should not create harm for yourself or those around you, which is why you are encouraged to pick a neutral person with integrity with whom to disclose your most personal thoughts, feelings, and actions. There may even be past events that are better served by sharing with a professional, such as a therapist, than a sponsor. We are guided to release secrets in order to set ourselves free; however, nowhere does it say that only one person has to know every secret.

Once you share the Fifth Step with a trusted someone, that person will be able to help identify your character qualities, both defects and assets. This is where integrity in action comes into play. This step cannot be worked alone.

When I first entered the residential treatment center it was imperative to find a sponsor right away in order to be in compliance with the treatment plan set forth. I didn't really want to talk to anybody, let alone ask a complete stranger to be my sponsor. Relying on my peers in the rehab center to give me the courage to trudge through the task of finding a sponsor, and to literally hold my hand while I choked on the words, "*Will you be my sponsor?*" yielded success. With my posse at my side, I psyched myself up that a particular night would be the night I would find a sponsor at the large meeting we were to attend, only because I felt I had no other options and was desperate, not because I was brimming with enthusiasm and willingness.

As I mentioned, integrity is important, but as a newcomer I didn't really care about integrity. I just didn't want to be thrown out of treatment for not following the rules because I had nowhere else to go. So, on this auspicious evening, as I gazed around the 12 Step meeting taking in the two hundred or more people in attendance, I quickly ruled out anyone I guessed was over forty, zeroed in on one of the younger women present, and decided she was a good candidate because her shoes and her earrings matched her outfit. I'm going to date myself, and this was not my usual genre, but picture ZZ Top's *"Legs"* video. Her outfit was right out of the video, complete with a tight mini skirt, lacy bobby socks worn with stilettos, and big earrings to top it off. Again, I was impressed that it all matched, so in my eyes she seemed qualified to sponsor. I asked her to sponsor me without even knowing her name, and she said yes. You may pause here to google search the ZZ Top video if desired.

An auspicious evening it was indeed, because I could go on and on about the lessons I learned from this woman. The most unexpected revelation of all is that once you get past appearances, we are all the same. As our relationship developed, I learned that she was raised very differently from me in regards to circumstance and culture. In fact, she was raised in what is historically known as a third world country in Asia, and our backgrounds were nothing alike. Even in our addiction we looked different. She had an education, worked hard, and was a professional, and I was a vagabond with a job, who threw away opportunity. Regardless of upbringing or background, no matter where we come from, at our core we all share similar feelings. When I shared my Fifth Step with her, she looked at me and simply stated she had the very same feelings in her addiction and in her recovery. She understood me, and that was enough for the healing to begin.

The yogic limb of *Niyama*, specifically self-study and reflection through *Svadhyaya*, fosters the development of personal values and integrity through connection to spirit. It's an inside job, but not a solo journey. Relationships provide the opportunity to more clearly see the self. Underneath the surface of the individual selves, we are connected like the threads in a spider's web, strong and purposeful while almost completely invisible. The essence of yoga is union. Together we walk the road of life, easing each other's burdens and sharing each other's joys. We are different expressions of one humanity.

Testimonial:

"A shared burden is lighter. To me, the Fourth and Fifth Chakras speak to the Fifth Step of AA. To do the Fifth, you have to open your heart (Fourth Chakra, truth and feeling) and unburden yourself to another person (Fifth Chakra, communication and purification). It is a fantastic experience! But challenging, just like Kundalini Yoga. You have to stretch yourself for recovery, just as for yoga (literally!). I learned that yoga means yoke from my teacher, Patty. That refers to connection – connection with the higher consciousness of the cosmos, connection with the teachers and yogis who brought the ideas of yoga forward in time, and connection with each other whenever we are practicing yoga and meditation (even if we are alone – because we're not alone!). If you want to recover in AA, you have to connect to others, too, especially when we are doing something like the 5ᵗʰ Step with our sponsor. You have to eventually connect with your Higher Power, and of course with the community in every meeting. We still learn from people long dead and feel a kinship with everyone who has helped bring their ideas into the present." - Puran Kaur

Bonus:

Guided Meditation

"Meditate on an attachment you would like to be rid of, an addiction or dependence you have. Visualize yourself walking across a landscape toward a place you want to be. There is a rope tied to you and on the other end is a box carrying the attachment. You take a knife and cut the rope, making the conscious decision to let go of the attachment. This is a turning point. The rest of the walk is easier now that you have let go of the attachment." -Barbara Ann Kipfer, *Natural Meditation* (2018)

Yoga Recommendation:

Step Five is deserving of cooling and calming energy. *Sitali Pranayam* helps in releasing anger, as it literally cools the body and a hot temper. This breath can be practiced for a few minutes anytime throughout the day.

Sitali Pranayam

Sit in a comfortable meditative posture with a straight spine. Curl the tongue up on the sides and protrude it slightly past the lips. (In California we call this a taco tongue.) Inhale deeply and smoothly through the rolled tongue and exhale through the nose. Continue for 5 minutes. Inhale, hold, pull the tongue in and relax. Then repeat for 5 more minutes.

Variations include: 2 to 3 minute periods, and the practice of 52 breaths daily, 26 in the morning and 26 at night.

Sitali Pranayam is a well-known practice. It soothes and cools the spine near the 4th, 5th, and 6th vertebrae, which, in turn, regulates the sexual and digestive energy. This breath is often used for lowering fever, and it can cool you in warm weather. Daily practice of 26 breaths in the morning and 26 breaths in the evening is said to extend the lifespan. The tongue may taste bitter at first, a sign of toxification, but as you continue the tongue will taste sweet and you will overcome sickness inside.

It is said that people who practice this kriya have all things that they need come to them by planetary ether. In mystical terms, you are served by the heavens.

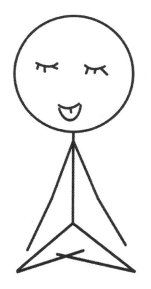

Author note:

If your tongue does not curl up on the sides, simply extend the tongue out slightly over the lips and practice the breath this way.

13

Step Six

"We were entirely ready to have God remove all these defects of character."

"What we must recognize is that we exult in some of our defects. Self-righteous anger can be very enjoyable. In a perverse way we can actually take satisfaction from the fact that many people annoy us; it brings a comfortable feeling of superiority." -Bill Wilson (1967)

What is a character defect and why do we need to ready ourselves for their removal? If these survival techniques have served to protect us, why can't we keep them? It's time to move beyond simple survival to authenticity.

We can't keep them because we have been misusing our emotions, and not listening to the wisdom of our feelings. In active addiction we have not been true to ourselves. We need to return to awareness and willingness to begin Step Six.

In a single sentence, what Step Six revealed to me is that my perceived assets were actually liabilities, and what I considered liabilities were actually assets. I had to make a complete 180 degree turn in the way I interpreted my thinking and my tendency to behave. For instance, I believed that being emotionally closed off and totally self-sufficient was an asset, I don't have to let anyone in, I can take care of myself, don't ask for help and I won't be rejected. This was all done unconsciously, in an attempt to avoid being hurt. Or at the very minimum I could portray this on the outside, so no one would actually see the vulnerable, crumbling inside. I thought the ability to shut down and not show emotion was an asset, so conversely, expressing emotion or weakness, or needing help was viewed as a liability. I quickly learned I needed to let people in, express feelings, and ask for help. What I needed most for my overall well-being was something I had been denying for most of my life. I had to switch my thought process and change my understanding of assets and liabilities.

On a side note, like it or not, the "I am an island" attitude, and the insistence to "do it all by myself" is actually an expression of feeling unworthy.

We are asked to be willing to look at our defects of character, or liabilities, so that we may move beyond them. We actually make a written list of them so we can make an effort to be honest about our thoughts, motives, and behaviors, and look at how we want to make changes. For instance, instead of attempting to be completely self-sufficient, with an "I don't need you" attitude, I open myself to others' love and help. The idea is simple, but it doesn't come as a natural default just because we've read the step and identified some of our own liabilities. It takes awareness and effort to get ready to put this new way of living into practice. We begin to realize that our behavior is a reflection of ourselves, not others. Step Six prepares us to move beyond our ordinary distractions and reactions. Writing our list of defects is the action prescribed to get us ready to have defects removed.

"So often in life, things that you regard as an impediment turn out to be great, good fortune."-Ruth Bader Ginsburg

One of the biggest challenges may be to identify defects of character. Any behavior, attitude, or thought that separates you from others, or supports isolation and the feeling of terminal uniqueness, is probably a character defect. Some sponsors in the program suggest to those they sponsor to begin by looking at the seven deadly sins, and then exploring how behavior manifests from this list of seven. The seven deadly sins are envy, gluttony, greed, lust, pride, sloth, and wrath. I have not included this to imply or weigh in on the concept of sin, but to give a beginning point for identifying character defects. If you prefer, you can look up lists of defects numbering beyond one hundred, but quite frankly I find those to be overly redundant and repetitive.

To keep it simple, what we need to know is how we act when we feel jealous, greedy, superior or inferior, lazy, hurt, or angry. How we protect ourselves when we feel vulnerable or exposed offers a window into our character defects.

The bottom line is a defect of character is anything that separates you from your true being, anything that blocks you from acting from the soul body, anything that denies your spiritual nature. When we act in a way that goes against who we really are, it harms our character and can be seen as a shortcoming.

There may be cases, for whatever reason, when we have been forced to behave in a manner that we would not naturally choose in order to survive. The example that comes readily to mind is from a client I worked with years ago. He struggled with defining personal defects of character versus accepting full responsibility for actions taken in the name of duty while serving in the armed forces. As a young person in the Vietnam War, actions were taken in compliance with official government orders and for survival that were not in accord with personal values and beliefs. The challenge here was to take responsibility for behavior, without continuing to judge and punish the self for actions taken outside of the realm of personal command. The war-time experience went on the Step Six list of defects because, in fact, it had harmed the pure human spirit of this individual. However, in this case the new behavior called for was self-forgiveness. Step Six is an evaluation of character to determine what defects played a part and when, what you want to change, and what you may have been holding yourself accountable for that was beyond your control. This step is all about preparation. In becoming entirely ready to have defects of character removed, clarity is essential.

People around you may unwittingly help to provide clarity. You may have heard the saying "*if you spot it, you've got it,*" and this certainly rings true when we're talking about character defects. The person who pushes your buttons, rubs you the wrong way, or maybe you simply dislike something about them, is actually reflecting an aspect of you back to yourself. This can be helpful in identifying your own defects of character. Yoga directs us to remember that the other person is us. The step refers to being ready to ask God to remove the defects, but it's the community around you that offers insight and support in this process. Yes, it's a process. If you haven't picked up on the theme of recovery yet, it's all a process. Step Six is not a one and done step, it's an ongoing relationship with willingness and a call to change.

Willingness is the key to this step. Being willing and doing the work of recovery is not always pretty. The outer mask, how we look to others, may need to be sacrificed in order to save the whole person. This brings me to the notion that yoga is not about getting a tight ass, it's about getting your head out of it. When I need to get my head on straight, a vigorous yoga set helps me to reset by clearing out old, residual thoughts and emotions, and making room for fresh input.

Yoga assists in the balancing of *prana* and *apana*, what we take in and what we release. When *apana* is balanced in the body, there is a greater inner knowing of what qualities are serving us well and what qualities we need to let go of. Identifying what we need to let go of through Step Six allows us to learn to walk lighter on the earth.

Once a list of personal defects of character is completed, it is recommended to share it with the person who received your Fifth Step, probably your sponsor, because they will help you with clarity, and maybe even add a few items to your list of defects.

Testimonial:

"I found yoga a good many years into recovery and it provided the tools to stay awake. The mind is a tricky thing; it is so fast and diverse. Yet it is one of our most powerful tools. When

it is focused and pointed in the right direction, we come to life. When undirected, it can lead us down some real rabbit holes. Substance abuse, habitually bad relationship choices, overconsumption of food or shopping, mindless scrolling, low self-esteem – we all know the list." - Anonymous

Bonus:

Espom Salt Soak

Add 1 ½ cups of Epsom Salt to a warm bath and soak in the tub. Add a few drops of pure essential oil, such as lavender for calming, if desired. Soaking in salt water helps to heal dark energy and sadness, and restore balance. It also aids the body in better mineral absorption.

Yoga Recommendation:

In Steps Six and Seven the work is done on the inside and the outside. The principle of willingness and a sense of coming into the self is present in these steps and in the fifth chakra. Assessment, action, and expression are key. The meditation for habituation is recommended for the positive benefits, both internal and external.

Habituation Meditation

Sit in Easy Pose with a straight spine, making sure that the first six lower vertebrae are locked forward. Make fists with both hands and extend the thumbs straight. Place the thumbs on the temples, and find the niche where the thumbs fit just right.

Lock the back molars together and keep the lips closed. The molars will alternately tighten, then release; right then left, then right and so on. You should feel the alternating movement under the thumbs at the temples. Keep a firm pressure applied on the temples. Keep the mouth closed, focus at the brow point, and mentally hear the sound of *Sa Ta Na Ma*, one sound for each pressing of the molars. Continue coordinating the mantra with subtle movement of the jaws for 5 to 7 minutes. With practice the time can be increased to 20 minutes, and ultimately 31 minutes.

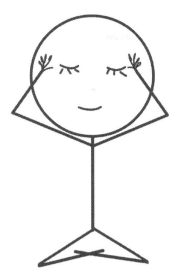

The imbalance in the pineal area upsets the pulsation of the pineal gland itself. It is this pulsation that regulates the pituitary gland, which regulates the rest of the glands. As the glands go, so follows the body and mind, thus creating an imbalance that results in unhealthy habits or addiction.

The pressure exerted by the thumbs triggers a rhythmic current into the central brain. This current activates the brain area directly under the stem of the pineal gland, helping to restore balance. It is an excellent meditation for the rehabilitation process in addictions and mental imbalances, as well as for breaking unwanted habits, such as smoking, drinking, and overeating.

To break unhealthy or unwanted habits there must be a change in the brain chemistry. According to the yogic science, mental and physical addictions are created by an imbalance around the stem of the pineal gland in the center of the brain.

14

Step Seven

"We humbly asked Him to remove our shortcomings."

"Of course, I slip up on a daily basis, mid-interaction I think, "hang on, I'm being totally selfish here," but I only have this awareness because I work this program. I have a template." -Russell Brand (2017)

The character defects that have been identified in Step Six will now be referred to as shortcomings in Step Seven. The two descriptions, character defects and shortcomings, may be used interchangeably. Defects listed and investigated, we now, with sincere humility, ask for these shortcomings to be removed. This concept of asking for removal refers directly to prayer. If you're still struggling to develop a relationship with a Higher Power, or God of your understanding, don't let this stop you in moving forward. If needed, simply return to willingness and open-mindedness to walk through any hesitation.

Humility is the principle of Step Seven. Being humble and having humility is much different than humiliation. Humiliation can ignite feelings of shame and loss of dignity. Being humble is a proactive approach to standing in our own truth. Humility is about having your feet on the ground, and neither inflating or deflating personal attributes. Humility ties into truth and resonates with neutrality found in the heart center.

Step Seven is short and sweet. It says to ask. Very much as in Step Three, Step Seven also implies an action, a letting go of results, and plenty of footwork to follow. Identifying the negative consequence of each shortcoming may encourage an earnest desire to change. Feeling the pain, isolation, and harm created by the shortcoming may actually help to create the humility needed to ask for assistance in releasing old, largely automatic, destructive patterns. The follow-up involves making a conscious choice to behave differently, for instance substituting acceptance in place of judgement.

A couple of years into recovery I was privy to an ongoing story from a co-worker who began praying for patience in an attempt to work on his impatience. He was finding his impatience and temper to be a problem for him and started to pray daily for patience.

He did this religiously for weeks, waiting for patience to be granted from above. A couple weeks into this process he began to complain that he was praying for patience, but instead found that his patience was being tried everywhere he went. For example, he found himself in line at the supermarket behind a woman with multiple children hanging noisily off the cart, using a large stack of coupons and paying with a check, and he reported regularly hitting every red light on this daily travels. The more he prayed for patience, the more he found his patience being challenged. He continued with his daily prayer, asking for patience, and still found himself in challenging situations. Another week or so into the process the light bulb went on for him, and he realized he was being given the opportunity to develop patience. It wasn't a quality that was going to hit and infuse him like a bolt of light from the sky, but rather something he would be able to develop in his own character through practice. By encountering these provoking experiences and not acting out by being rude to others or storming off, but rather waiting patiently through them, he was able to develop patience within himself. This is a great example of how we learn through experience, many times experience involving obstacles or challenges. As my co-worker's patience story came to an end, his biggest message was to be careful what you pray for because you just might get it, and it may not be on your own terms.

The powerful message of this story has never left me, and I have also never prayed for patience. My prayers are more along the line of requesting alignment with God's will, and letting go. I realize it's my responsibility to develop my character, and the universe provides plenty of opportunities for this type of growth without me asking for extra lessons.

Shortcomings can be silently sneaky or out loud in your face. Sometimes they start out quiet and build in intensity, until they cannot be ignored. Being judgmental is one of my personal, glaring defects of character and it recurs even decades into recovery. I cannot tell you how many times unfairly, secretly, judging another has come back to bite me in the behind and dish up a whopping serving of humble pie. This shortcoming is very different than simply using sound judgement in our daily lives, like not walking alone on a dark street at night, because it has no base in reality or truth. It is fictional, negative judgment that creates a divide, a feeling of superiority, and a separation or isolation from others. A pattern of negative consequences may run a similar course with any of our character defects. I've mentioned earlier in this book that our thoughts do not always represent our true self. The good news is that perfection is not required for recovery, and the choice to continue to evolve and work on the self is always an option.

In asking for shortcomings to be removed, Step Seven also allows for the circumventing of destructive behavior, meaning the self-correction may be made prior to acting out the negative behavior. The external response and reaction pattern may be changed. Step Seven may also be seen as an invitation to cease looking for opportunities to be offended.

"Taking a moment to figure out how you really feel instead of letting old patterns decide for you is one of the most authentic things you can do." - Yung Pueblo (2021)

The yogic principles found in the *Yamas,* or restraints, align well with Step Seven. The restraints are a recommended practice in order to avoid harmful behaviors and attitudes, and are the base for walking the yogic journey. When we practice *asana, pranayam,* and meditation on a regular basis we direct movement of the body in a way so that the construction of these principles begins to solidify in our being. We stretch and open into something new on a physical, mental, and emotional level.

Testimonial:

"Meditation is incredibly challenging for anyone let alone someone in recovery with a case of the monkey mind. Kundalini yoga has helped to dispel the myth that meditation is unobtainable. Kundalini has helped me to break patterns I thought I would never be able to process, let alone let go of. Letting go is a difficult process and you hear this in meetings, but how does one let go of something? Kundalini yoga has been that action for me." - Tracy T.

Bonus:

Laughing Activity

Find ways to laugh today. Whether in groups of people or by yourself, spontaneous or forced, take time to laugh today. Along with the below benefits of laughter, it is also helps us not take ourselves so seriously.

"Laughter lowers the flow of dangerous stress hormones that suppress the immune system, raise blood pressure, and increase the number of platelets, which cause clots and potentially fatal coronary artery blockages. Laughter also eases digestion and soothes stomachaches, a common symptom of chronic stress. Plus, a good rollicking guffaw increases the release of endorphins, which makes you feel better and more relaxed. Laughter truly may be the best medicine when it comes to stress relief." – Dr. Daniel Amen, Change Your Brain, Change Your Body (2010)

Yoga Recommendation:

Anti-Stress Breathing is the very practical recommendation for Step Seven. Doing things differently can be stressful, and this is an easy practice to counter both old and new stressors.

<u>Anti-Stress Breathing</u>

In meditation posture, press tips of the thumbs and little fingers together. The other fingers touch each other on the same hand, but do not touch the opposite fingers, and are extended straight out between the navel and the heart center with the arms comfortably relaxed at the sides. Eyes focus at the tip of the nose.

Inhale through the mouth with a long, deep and powerful breath, and exhale through the nose. Then inhale through the nose and exhale through the mouth. Continue this cycle for 11 minutes. It is recommended to do this meditation for 90 days. Balances the pituitary so that you don't receive every bit of information. Calms inner tension.

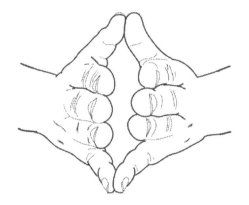

15

Step Eight

"We made a list of all persons we had harmed, and became willing to make amends to them all."

"When we begin just to try to accept ourselves, the ancient burden of self-importance lightens up considerably." -Pema Chodron (1997)

Yeah, but…, what about what they did to me? Nope, sorry, it doesn't matter what the other person has done. Step Eight is about cleaning up your side of the street by identifying who, or what, you have harmed. It also indicates we become willing to make amends, not that we are making amends. Leave Step Nine alone for now.

Quite literally we make a list of those harmed, including people and places, and take care to make sure the list is complete. People may be family, friends, employers, co-workers, enemies, or strangers that have been harmed in the course of our addiction. Beyond identifying individual persons there may be places frequented that were harmed, such as the workplace, drinking or gambling establishments, retail stores, the local park or event arenas, etc. This is simply a list, not a commitment. General offensive behavior in public places may be listed in a blanket statement; however, I recommend personal relationships each get their own mention on the list. Each relationship will elicit its own emotion.

For instance, it may be quite emotionally distressing to list loved ones who have been the recipient of hurtful, negligent, or unwanted behavior and to actually identify the harm inflicted. Whereas, being the obnoxious drunk who pissed off the whole camp ground by keeping them up at night may cause a twinge of mild regret, especially compared to damage caused in intimate relationships. You can draw on the experience of writing and sharing your Fourth Step inventory to help write the Eighth Step list.

It is also important to note that the severity of the harm may not necessarily be directly proportionate to the guilt, shame, or remorse felt about the behavior. This is similar to trauma in that the severity of the trauma does not always reflect proportionately to the outward response. Sometimes we respond to a gentle lapping tide as if it is a tsunami, or vice versa. Remember we just learned from Step Seven that judging is not in our best interest, and that includes deciding how bad someone should or should not feel, including ourselves.

For example, I had a co-worker on my list of amends. He was a quiet, polite man I had worked with for a few years while waiting tables at a local restaurant. Since cash was readily available from tips, I borrowed $20 from him one night and never paid him back. I would think about it every time I looked at him, and knew he knew, but he was too kind to say anything so I never squared up. If I coughed up the money to pay him back, I would lack money for my next fix, so I pretended I forgot. Honestly, I've done way worse things than this and not given them a second thought, but this one bothered me. Make a complete list, regardless of perceived severity of harm. If it comes to your awareness, write it down!

Make sure to put yourself on your list too! Left to my own devices this never would have occurred to me. Thankfully we don't work the steps alone, so there was someone there to remind me that I count, too. We do harm ourselves, and we have the opportunity to look at how we want to make these amends to self.

A friend recently pointed out an unexpected and added advantage of writing down and evaluating an Eighth Step list. The advantage she shared is an increased openness to accepting others' apologies and giving other people a second chance, just as that opportunity has been extended to her in recovery.

The principle of Step Eight is responsibility. Whether we are the identified addict or the co-dependent who works hard to try to manage a loved one who is deemed out of control, we again have to look at ourselves honestly in this step. Whatever the harmful fixation we become entangled in, either knowingly or unknowingly, we find we now have the power to identify the behavior, relationships, and situations we wish to amend. The below story, although written as fiction, is based on the author's life experience and demonstrates how change can evolve from the courage of taking one small action.

Crystal Rainbows

Susan gazed at the single teardrop crystal hanging in her kitchen window reflecting the late afternoon sun. She wondered how something so small could scatter such brilliant rainbows across an entire room. And do so with such color and splendor. Then she thought it is often the smallest of things, or gestures or deeds that are the catalysts for grander events to follow.

As Susan continued to gaze at the crystal her mother had given her, her thoughts went to a time some five years past. She had gone to visit the mother she had not seen in twelve years. She was at the same time terrified and elated.

As Susan passed the boarding gates and walked toward the airport exit, she caught sight of a slight and elderly looking woman she recognized. The years had not been kind to this woman.

The lines and creases cast shadows across her face as tears spilled from her eyes. But she was smiling. The biggest smile Susan had ever seen her mother possess.

With a sigh, Susan then knew the years would melt away and love would be restored. Susan startled herself to the present. She flicked the crystal to catch more of the sunlight. It swayed gently to and fro as if to say, "Yes, this is the beginning of the story, right, not the ending." Yes, she thought, this was only the beginning of a whole new chapter. Susan decided she still had time before preparing the evening meal to indulge herself in a few minutes of quiet reminiscing. So, after pouring herself a cup of coffee, moving to the family room and settling into her favorite chair, her thoughts again drifted backwards in time.

It seemed like a lifetime ago. Her mother divorcing her 4th husband and becoming addicted to pills again. Susan shuddered at the thought of the pills and alcohol her mother consumed. Her mother said it eased her pain, but Susan knew it only created more pain. In such an angry bewildered state, her mother would strike out at anyone and everyone around. Susan knew this first hand. It was the reason for the long separation. Her mother had finally driven Susan away with the cruel comments and threats that did not bear thinking about again.

Then, Susan remembered how five years ago she had finally decided to write one last letter to her mother. A letter filled with honesty, doubt, hope, despair, and love. A letter she dared not hope would be answered. But it was answered by a short letter from her mother; followed by another. Then came a brief phone conversation. Susan remembered how each of them had chosen their words so carefully. One phone call led to another until finally Susan decided to make a trip to Idaho to visit her mother.

Susan quickly flashed through the happiness of the first trip, the ongoing phone calls, the cards and letters, the second trip, and the third. She recalled the happy shopping excursions they made together. She laughed to herself about all the "bargain" treasures they had purchased and the lunches filled with laughter and lively conversation. A tear slid down Susan's cheek as she recalled her mother's apology. It wasn't long, nor was it elegant, but it was sincere. Her mother had simply said, "Susan, I am truly sorry for all the pain and heartache I have caused you. Please accept my apology." Susan remembered how she could barely nod her head in acknowledgement of this apology. She knew her mother was never one to apologize. The apology had been very hard for her mother to verbalize. And it had meant the world to Susan.

She looked up to see that the crystal had stopped swaying, the sun had disappeared behind the trees, and it was definitely time to start the evening meal. Arising from her favorite chair Susan smiled to herself. Even though no one was around she said out loud: "Thank heavens for the little things in life that come to bring so much change."

As Susan was heading toward the kitchen the phone began to ring. She picked up the receiver and heard her mother's voice on the other end of the line. "Hello, Mother. Yes, I was just thinking about you too. You remember the crystal you gave me five years ago? It still looks beautiful in the window. Thank you again so very much. Yes, I think we will have a white Christmas in Idaho again this year. I'm really looking forward to it too. See you the day after tomorrow. Love you too. Bye." After replacing the phone Susan looked at the crystal again and said, more to it than herself, "May everyone be so blessed with such brilliant rainbows. - Peggy H.

In my first book, *Yogable,* I talk about approaching the practice of yoga with *Ahimsa* which translates as non-harming. We can apply this principle to Step Eight and to life; moving forward in recovery with compassion, tolerance, and kindness for ourselves as well as others.

Testimonial:

"Kundalini Yoga is what I call the direct jet-route to self acceptance." -Polly S.

Bonus:

<u>An Apology Practice Quiz</u>

In preparation for Step Nine, where actual apologies may be made, as well as identifying amends, let's take a look at how to say "I'm sorry" in a respectful way. Please read the list of various apologies and choose all of the appropriate options.

   a. I'm sorry, but I was in my addiction and wasn't able to make better choices.
   b. I'm sorry if I hurt you during my addiction.
   c. I'm sorry I caused harm to you and betrayed your trust.
   d. I'd like to apologize for what I said, but that's just how I talk to everyone, you know I didn't really mean it.
   e. I apologize for hurting you and I take full responsibility for my actions while I was drinking and using.
   f. I was dishonest with you. I extend my apology, and plan to make amends to you by practicing honesty in our relationship.

The correct options are c, e, and f. Anytime a "but" or "if" is added it negates the apology. It simply wipes it right out. Minimizing or rationalizing, saying that's "just how I am" is also an excuse, not an apology. Be honest, direct, and keep it simple.

Yoga Recommendations:

The fifth chakra is still front and center for Steps Eight and Nine as they employ clear vision, maturity, and the actual use of the voice. When working these steps, a balanced fifth chakra gives courage to speak the truth and moderation in not saying too much or too little. (Think of Baby Bear's porridge in the story of Goldilocks, not too cold or hot, but just right.) Yoga for Drug Damage and a meditation for depression and the brain are practices given to begin repairing actual damage to the body and mind from active addiction.

Simple stretch to warm-up the 5th chakra. This also works the muscles and skin of the neck and face. Sit in Rock Pose, tilt the chip up and blow kisses toward the sky. Practice for 20 seconds, relax, and repeat 2 more times.

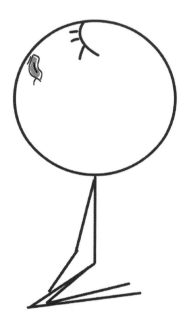

Yoga for Drug Damage

1. Lie down on your back, with hands in Venus Lock behind the neck, raise straight legs up to 24" off the ground and hold with Long Deep Breathing for 3 minutes.

2. Still on your back, raise legs to ninety degrees, inhale and spread them wide out to each side, exhale and bring them together. Repeat and continue for 3 minutes.

3. Still on your back, bring the knees to the chest, wrap arms around the legs and roll back and forth along the length of the spine for 3 minutes.

4. In Rock Pose, sitting on the heels, place hands on the ground 8" before the knees. Inhale, exhale and bend forward placing the forehead on the floor. Inhale up and exhale down for 3 minutes. Alternate with Easy Pose or sit with legs extended if Rock Pose puts too much pressure on the knees.

5. Still in Rock Pose, place hands in Venus Lock above the head and chant Hum, Hum, Hum for 3-11 minutes. Hum means "We the total Universe." Let the word Hum be chanted as though humming as you draw out the vibration.

Relax in Corpse Pose on the back.

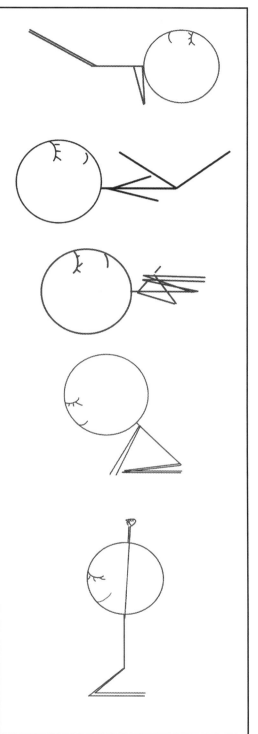

Anti-Depression & Brain Synchrony Meditation

For Former Marijuana Users (good for everyone!)

In Easy Pose with a straight spine, raise the upper arms parallel to the ground, hands in Gyan Mudra. Raise mudras in front of the eyes, and stare through them with wide open eyes, beyond the hands to the horizon. Inhale deeply as you separate the hands 36-45 inches out to the sides, while keeping the eyes fixed on the horizon. Exhale back to the original position. Keep the elbows relaxed. One cycle takes about 4 seconds. As the hands go out, mentally vibrate "Sa," as they return, "Ta," out "Na," return "Ma," and so on. Meditate on the life energy in the breath. The mental feeling of stretching the breath from a single point to the width of the arm spread is essential. After 2-3 minutes, increase speed to 3 ½ to 4 seconds for each cycle of "Sa Ta Na Ma," and continue for 3 more minutes. Then inhale and relax, arms and shoulders are totally dead. No mudra is needed, just RELAX. Or meditate at the crown chakra, and focus all your energy at the anterior fontanel on top of the skull. Put all of your energy into total relaxation or on that one square inch on the skull. Continue about 15 minutes.

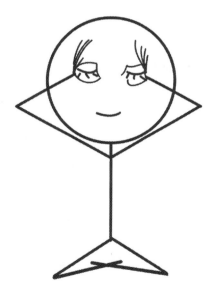

Comments: You were born to be positive and creative. The creativity of your existence is unlimited. Since we have not established the habit of constancy in thought and action, we create negative patterns of thought and depression. This meditation will let you evaluate and measure how positive or negative you are and it will make you positive and happy. It focuses on the range of the breath. In the subconscious, breath and life are synonymous. By meditating this way, depression can be alleviated. If done correctly, there will be pressure at the lymph glands. The two sides of the brain are separated and coordinated.

Those who used marijuana at any time in their life get the hemispheres confused. The effect is periodic scatteredness, lack of motivation, depression or alienation. This can recur anytime in life, even after years of abstinence. This exercise will also re-coordinate the brain functions. Increase the time of the meditation slowly. Ultimately you can do it for 11 minutes, followed by the relaxation of 31 minutes.

16

Step Nine

"We made direct amends to such people wherever possible, except when to do so would injure them or others."

"Guilt is an internal compass that uses mistakes to teach responsibility and integrity. This strict internal judge guides you to be true to your Self." - GuruMeher Khalsa (2013)

Eighth Step list complete, we now move to Step Nine. Typically, this list is shared and reviewed with a sponsor for guidance. We don't get to decide willy-nilly who we're going to make amends to and how to proceed on our own. This step is taken with direction so that amends are made in a way that may be most beneficial, and safe, for the receiver and the giver. Amends are not the equivalent to apologizing or saying *"I'm sorry,"* but rather taking responsibility and creating a plan for change. In the process of making amends an apology may be fitting in the owning of harmful behavior and the desire to clean up the wreckage of the past, but remember to amend is to change. We can ask ourselves, what needs to be repaired and what's going to be different if we are to resume relationships with those we have hurt. An opportunity is available to choose a possibly uncomfortable, honest conversation instead of holding on to the past. In the long run silence is more costly. It takes discipline to show up and face those we hurt.

In addition to taking responsibility for our actions, we employ discipline for ongoing maintenance. Discipline is needed to remain willing to be accountable for all of our actions, and to follow through on implementing changes in behavior.

Fantasies and ideas of making amends ran through my head before going over my list with my sponsor, and when we got down to it, she burst my bubble. She completely called me out and exposed my underlying motives. I guess she was listening during Step Five. First of all, she told me a simple apology to my family members was not going to be sufficient. She told me I was going to make what are called living amends. In making living amends I was directed to show up clean and sober, be present, and interact honestly with my family in the days and years to come. That's exactly what I've done for three decades. I've not been the perfect daughter, sister, wife, or mother, but I show up and am accountable for my behavior, even when I mess up.

An ex-boyfriend was on the list, too, and I was eager to contact him to make amends and maybe introduce him to the program, you know, maybe suggest a meeting and help him get clean. The last time I saw him we were fighting over a hypodermic needle in the middle of a quiet residential street. He said it was his, and I knew it was mine. He took it and ran off and I'd had no contact since. Certainly, I owed his mother amends too. Well, my dear sponsor told me that what he and his family were up to was none of my business and that my amends to them was to stay out of their lives, and to not cause disruption. She saw through the weak veil of my ulterior motive and told me to stay the hell away from him and his family. I thought, "I'm so sure, like I'm the problem?" She was, of course, right on target for my overall wellbeing.

The universe works in mysterious ways. Twenty some years later the ex-boyfriend mentioned above surfaced on social media. It turned out we lived in the same city and our kids ended up in the same school. He was clean in the program too. Amends were made on both sides with peaceful resolution and forgiveness.

Ignoring amends that need to be made does not make them go away. At my twenty-year high school reunion, I finally made an amends I had previously chickened out of due to fear of the response. It may not have been a big deal to her, but it never went away for me. I had to say the words out loud in order to clean my side of the street.

Prayer and positive intention went out to those I was unable to contact directly. I was not able to locate my fellow waiter from the previous chapter, so instead of returning the $20, I prayed for his prosperity. I still do whenever I think about it.

What we don't get to do is assuage our guilt or relieve our conscience at the expense of others. So, no running out to confess to your best friend that you had an affair with their spouse. You don't have to throw yourself on the front steps of the courthouse for minor infractions. However, you can shop at places you stole from and spend honest dollars earned in establishments you cheated, unless of course, these places will put you in the way of harm. If amends cannot be made directly, be creative in working with your sponsor to plan realistic actions that can be taken with the intent to repair past damage. Some ideas include throwing extra cash in the basket at meetings or church, or giving of your time to charitable organizations.

We don't get to avoid amends because they will be uncomfortable, but we do account for our safety. Friends in Alanon have shared a saying that goes something like this, *"Say what you mean, mean what you say, but don't say it mean."* There's no need to cause more harm by being brutally honest. This is a step of reparation, so please take this into consideration and act accordingly. No guarantees are given that our amends will be accepted, so we want to approach each amend without expectation. If we go in thinking we will be immediately forgiven and the amends will end with a big hug, we may be sorely disappointed. The action called for in this step is best taken with the direction of a sponsor, and in the spirit of love and faith.

Amends to the self are made this way, too. We can make better choices to take care of ourself in a healthy way and be honest to the best of our ability as we interact with our internal and external environment. First and foremost, we can make amends to ourselves by showing up at 12 Step meetings and staying clean one more day.

We can also make amends to ourselves by engaging in healthy exercise, yoga, and meditation. Even in the rooms of recovery there is a large focus on mental, emotional, and spiritual growth, and the physical body sometimes gets ignored. Physical movement is essential for a balanced lifestyle. I feel so refreshed, relaxed and alive after practicing yoga. Entering this state on a regular basis aids in mental and emotional processing.

The following Step Ten closes a loop hole, so we don't slip through. We may continue to make amends as needed throughout recovery. The active learning process has taken place, now it's time for maintenance.

Testimonial:

"After being in recovery for 24 years I started doing Kundalini yoga. In recovery we are looking for mind, body, spirit balance and I can say this is the closest thing I've found to get there. Being post-menopausal and having a work-related injury, it became harder for me to do the yoga and workouts I used to do. Kundalini classes are helping me to understand the mind, body, spirit connection and balance. There's one thing that has stood out the most for me as a recovering addict, and that is to give yourself permission to relax!" -Denise H.

Bonus:

Gratitude Activity

"Here is a quick gratitude exercise you can try. Write down five things you are grateful for every day. The act of writing helps to solidify them in your brain. In my experience, when depressed patients did this exercise every day, they actually needed less antidepressant medication. Other researchers have also found that people who express gratitude on a regular basis are healthier, more optimistic, make more progress toward their goals, have a greater sense of well-being, and are more helpful to others. Practicing gratitude literally helps you have a brain to be grateful for." - Dr. Daniel Amen *(2010)*

For best results this exercise in gratitude should be done with and pen, or pencil, and paper. Typing on a keyboard does not have the same result. I recommend having a separate journal designated for daily gratitude lists; however, this is not required. The main thing is to commit to writing a daily list. Try it out for 90 days and see how it goes.

I intentionally placed this activity in Step Nine for two reasons. One, this type of activity is helpful in assessing our attitude in daily life, and two, it can be difficult to connect with gratitude on a meaningful level in early recovery. Newcomers may have an aversion to the word gratitude simply because it has been out of the range of personal experience. By the time we are actively making amends the experience of gratitude in recovery is usually on the radar.

Yoga Recommendation:

Pelvic Rotation is given for Step Nine as it is an excellent cleanse for the liver and an example of a simple action that can be with the intention of making amends to the self. This exercise is good for the liver and digestion, as well as flexibility in the spine. Plus, it feels fabulous. These are affectionately called liver rolls. The exercise may be done seated with the hands on the knees as described below, or by standing with the feet about 18 to 24 inches apart and the hands on the hips.

Pelvic Rotation

Sit in Easy Pose, hold on to the knees and rotate the torso on the pelvis moving the spine in a big circle. Find your own range of motion, make it slow and gentle if needed, and move with the breath; inhale and exhale with each rotation. Move in each direction for equal amounts of time, 1 to 3 minutes. This posture opens the flow of energy at the base of the spine.

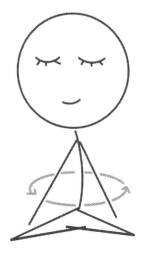

17

Step Ten

"We continued to take personal inventory and when we were wrong promptly admitted it."

"In reality it is much easier not to smoke or eat chocolate than to do so. It is your mind that convinces you otherwise." - Dr. Wayne W. Dyer (1993)

Having worked the previous nine steps, we now arrive at Step Ten. By this time we have usually gained enough personal insight to know when we are at fault or out of balance. Step Ten is about perseverance, and thus begins the maintenance portion of the program. It is not time to languish in the fruit of our labors from the preceding steps, but a time to maintain our forward momentum and growth. The first of the maintenance steps suggests taking a daily inventory, continuous self-reflection, and the righting of wrongs. We don't need to wait and accumulate a list of future amends to make because we are accountable for ourselves immediately. This step requires vigilance, so that we don't slip through the cracks. That being said, we most likely will slip through the cracks in attitude or behavior from time to time, but we don't have to stay there and it doesn't have to end in drinking, using, or acting out in addictive behaviors. Step Ten can be viewed as a safety net, or a filter, designed to catch destructive, defeating thoughts and behavior and self-correct as we continue in recovery.

If you're not sure what to review in your personal life, you can always go back and look at the reflection questions of the *yamas* and *niyamas* in Chapter 3.

Step Ten is worth some exploration. It can be done written formally, as a casual mental review, by meditation, or through discussion with a sponsor or trusted friend. As long as the strategy picked for Step Ten allows for an unbiased self-evaluation, it is acceptable.

A fairly recent conversation with a beloved friend shed light on the importance of being able to evaluate the self and embrace others from a neutral place. As I listened, the basic premise of the conversation that came my way went something along the lines of why change, because no one else does, and ultimately there's no reason to forgive others. What I heard from their sharing was a firm stance that change is an unreasonable response to pain and discomfort within relationships, and an absolute defending of emotional wounds and the right to be the victim. This stance is definitely an option. It's an option outside the realm of neutrality and healing, but an option nonetheless. A flippant remark was made that I am the only person she knows who has changed. I responded to that with a resounding yes, that's the point of life! Sometimes it feels as though my entire life is steeped in self-reflection. The steps and the yogic lifestyle describe taking responsibility for the self as the path to freedom and serenity, so yes, I am frequently evaluating my interaction with the world around me so that I can honestly determine how I am functioning on this earth. This allows me to identify changes I need to make so that I am comfortable in my own skin. I spend time in meditation, contemplation, journaling, and discussion regarding my life (feelings, attitude, and behavior) and how I affect those around me, as well as myself. At this point in my life, I am not only focusing and uncovering the negative aspects that need to be changed, but I can also identify what is working and what to keep. Again, I am by no means perfect in this pursuit, but I know that for my peace of mind I cannot afford to withhold forgiveness and remain a victim.

Although prior steps have already taken us through the work of beginning to forgive, both self and others, I want to elaborate on the concept of forgiveness here in Step Ten. The purpose of forgiveness is inner peace and healing. When we learn to forgive, we let ourselves off the hook of anger and resentment. It's actually not about the other person or situation that we are forgiving. I think society in general has a misguided idea of forgiveness. Most people I have worked with, in a professional and personal context, initially assume that it allows the perpetrator, perceived or real, off the hook and then all is just supposed to magically be well within the relationship. Forgiveness is actually extended as an act of letting go, not forgetting. We don't ever have to pursue a relationship with the person or situation being forgiven. We don't even have to like them. Forgiveness does not equate to a repairing of the relationship. If you are looking to reestablish a relationship with a loved one, it can and does happen, but is not the overall goal. Again, it's for our own healing and serenity. Forgiving from the heart center, rather than the head, allows clear boundaries to be established. Let the heart guide the way in all of your assessments and actions.

Consistent evaluation through personal inventory recently led me to make amends to a woman I sponsor for making negative comments about her husband. My intention was to validate her feelings, but the approach was off base. Originally, I did not realize the effect of my offhanded remarks, but when it did become apparent it was harmful, I owned it and changed the behavior. She laughed and dismissed it, but I knew I was wrong and took corrective action. This is a pretty straightforward example of righting wrongs as soon as they are revealed. (The rest of the women I sponsor are now all wondering who it was.)

Correcting self- destructive behavior can be more challenging because the nature of the disease is sneaky, and if we think we are not harming others the change needed is less obvious. Denial and minimization can arise at any time, which is why we have this step for ongoing vigilance.

Daily inventory can also keep us on track in regard to focusing on what is most important in our personal recovery so that we don't return to our old ways in thought or deed. Step Ten can help to keep our goals in the forefront of our consciousness at any stage of recovery. I'll use my husband and myself as an example. My husband and I met in long-term residential treatment. We had very little interaction to begin with, and over the course of nine months we became friends. Around this time, it was apparent that we were interested in dating, but it was prohibited due to our participation in the treatment center's staff training program. Quite frankly, in the past this would not have deterred either of us from doing whatever we wanted regardless of consequences. However, both of us knew that recovery was the priority, and as lame as it may seem, we were willing to follow direction and not date until after both of us had a year clean and we had moved out of the in-house training program. An additional motivating factor is that neither of us had anywhere to go, so it was in our best interest to finish the program so we could be employed and actually transition back into the community without being homeless. It may sound silly, but I sincerely believe we are still together today, over 30 years later, because we approached our relationship with honesty and the agreement that personal recovery comes first. Without personal recovery we wouldn't even have a relationship. Daily reflection in Step Ten supports commitment to recovery and the daily choices needed to follow through on that commitment by keeping our ego in check. We release the need for instant gratification. Stability can be maintained in spite of distraction.

Speaking of distraction, beware of taking another's inventory! We raised our children with the practice of regular personal inventory, without using those actual words, which leads to a funny story about my daughter becoming a party pooper. My daughter blasted one poor kid at a high school keg party when he claimed he was clean because he stopped using drugs and only drinks beer on the weekends. She told him verbatim, *"I don't know what program you're in, but in NA alcohol is a drug, so you're not clean."* She shared that in response, his face fell and he looked defeated. The moral of this story is that it's a good idea to avoid being too rigid in our unsolicited verbal assessments of others, and ourselves. However, here I will take the opportunity to openly share my objection to the newly coined term "California Sober." Any path of recovery that condones the use of mind or mood-altering chemicals is not in alignment with the Twelve Step principles and may be detrimental to those seeking real change and recovery. If you stop drinking, but smoke weed, you're not clean and sober. Psychiatric medications and treatment that is medically indicated by a physician may be excluded from the above blanket statement, as I am referring to recovery from recreational and self-medicating use of chemicals.

With perseverance, wrongs are revealed as recovery is maintained. We can self-correct when we veer off the path. Your inner voice will alert you to danger, just as your car may give a loud beep in warning when you inadvertently move out of your lane or get too close to another car. Tapping into the neutral mind through meditation helps intuition to reign. We may make repairs and restitution to ourselves and others when called for in daily life. It is truly a gift to have a clear conscience as the head hits the pillow each night.

Living life on life's terms in recovery imparts another beautiful discovery. The discovery of who we are; what we like, how we enjoy spending our time, and the ability to embrace our personal gifts, and our individual personality. We are given the privilege to extend the action of love to ourself and thus, build a fantastic future outside the grasp of active addiction.

Testimonial:

"When I get up in the morning and practice my 15 to 20 minute yoga routine, along with my daily 12 step practice, I feel relaxed and energized to start my day. I feel beautiful, well-rounded, and worthy of all the good things life has to offer." -Tina L.

Bonus:

Commit to keeping a nightly journal for 30 days, wherein you review each day in order to identify both personal strengths and weaknesses. This type of daily assessment will help you see what is working for you and what is not. You can write a few sentences or a few paragraphs. You get to choose to write as much or as little as desired, as long as you're reviewing your day in writing.

Yoga Recommendation:

The sixth chakra ties into intuition and the ability to listen to the inner voice. This powerful, but light hearted, *kriya* helps to not take the self so seriously while developing tolerance and acceptance. You will breathe, move, chant and laugh your way through awareness, tolerance and acceptance.

Handle Yourself/For Tolerance

This short set of exercises focuses on the solar plexus, your physical power center. It brings a quick boost to your confidence and self-control, and is therefore a good preparation for meditation. Use it as a daily practice to build a balanced use of your power. It can be done in 20 minutes at the full times listed, or reduce the times proportionately for a quicker lift. Take brief meditative rests between each exercise, or power right through for a more intense workout. Two cycles of the complete set will give you a good physical tune-up.

1. Sit comfortably on the floor with the spine upright yet relaxed. Curl the four fingers of both hands, then hook the right hand into the left with the right palm facing down. Push the side of the hands (right thumb knuckles) into your belly, just below the navel. Exhale completely and hold the breath out for 8 seconds with the abdomen holding firmly against the inward pressure of the hands. Then inhale and hold the breath for 8 seconds with the same two pressures. Continue this cycle for 3 minutes, then relax. Sit for a moment in calm self-awareness and feel your strength.

2. Sit on the heels, Rock Pose, and raise the arms overhead, pressing the palms flat together. Pull your navel in firmly as your powerfully utter "Sat" (pronounced more like "sut" in this instance). Then relax the navel as your calmly say "Nam." Continue for 3 minutes, then inhale and squeeze the entire body tightly for 5 to 15 seconds. Exhale, relax everything and sit quietly observing your sensations for 1 minute.

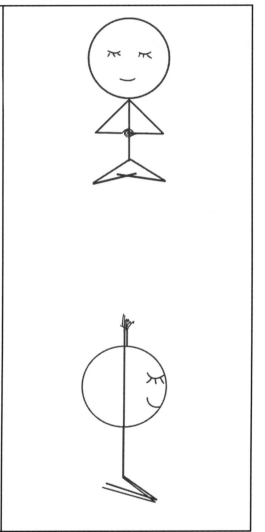

3. Stretch your legs out straight in front of you. Place the palms on the ground behind you. Raise both legs to 60 degrees and hold this position with a strong and steady Breath of Fire. Continue for 2 minutes, then inhale, exhale, and apply the Root Lock. Then relax immediately into Easy Pose and belly laugh loudly for 1 minute. Sit calmly in self-awareness.

4. In Easy Pose, bring your hands into fists at the shoulders. Inhale deeply and suspend the breath, then begin alternately punching forward as if boxing rapidly. When you must, exhale, and inhale deeply to continue. After 3 intense minutes, relax.

5. Still in Easy Pose, alternate between Camel Ride (Spinal Flex) and Shoulder Shrugs as follows. (a) Hold on to your ankles/shins and inhale as your flex the spine forward, then exhale- extend it back and (b) Inhale -lift the shoulders up to the ears, exhale – drop the shoulders down. Find your rhythm with the breath. The pace is about 5 full cycles in 10 seconds. Continue this cycle with deep breaths for 3 minutes. Then inhale, exhale completely, apply the Root Lock for as long as your like, then relax. Sit calmly and follow the sensations of energy and your own strength. Continue on to any meditation or move in to deep relaxation.

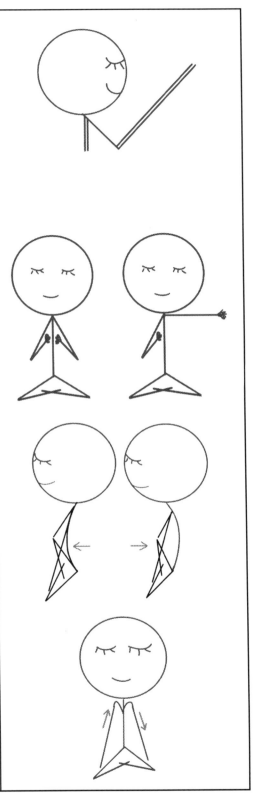

18

Step Eleven

"We sought through prayer and meditation to improve our conscious contact with God as we understood Him, praying only for knowledge of His will for us and the power to carry that out."

"Mind cannot be transcended by pursuing it, but only by the surrender of the illusion of mind as savior." -David R. Hawkins, MD, PhD (2011)

Meditation may be one of the most misunderstood aspects in all of the steps. Many believe the myth that in meditation we strive to stop the mind from thinking and sit in quiet bliss. Good luck with that! What we are building through Step Eleven is awareness. Meditation, as a part of that path, tunes us in, not shuts us down. The simplest explanation I have heard in the program is that prayer is asking, or sending out, and meditation is listening, or receiving. Ideally both come honestly from the heart center and there is no need to sugar coat communication with a Higher Power.

If we revisit previous chapters, you'll recall that the neutral mind is also referred to as the meditative mind and resides in the heart center. For prayer and meditation to be most effective, they must originate from a place of authenticity and sincerity. Even if you're just going through the motions to follow through on an original sincere desire, your efforts will be effective. There's no quantitative evaluation on your personal prayer or meditative life, you can do it just because it is suggested; your heart may not be in it to begin with, but let the action at least originate from a pure and honest willingness.

I can't tell you how many times I have sat through a meditation for ninety days, following through on the action because I made the original commitment, whether I wanted to each day or not. Some days I loved it and some days I hated it, but I reaped the benefits of my overall commitment regardless of how I felt about it on each individual day. My original intention was pure and I followed up with the footwork. Here we go with the footwork again!

Step Eleven is another maintenance step that does require action. It's more than simply reading the words and thinking that is sufficient to apply to life to actively work the step. It is taking the action of prayer and meditation that develops increased awareness, a necessity for ongoing recovery. No formal rite or format must be followed. Prayer and meditation are highly personal and intimate aspects of life. You can talk casually to your Higher Power or you can go to church and participate in familiar and comforting group worship. You can sit and meditate on the flow of your breath, follow guided meditation apps, join a meditation group, or engage in the more active type of meditations found in this book. All are simply suggestions, but let's be clear, it is suggested you try something. You get to decide what is right for you. Thank goodness Step One gave the gift of choice because you are empowered to use it again here in Step Eleven.

The step does state that we are asking for knowledge of His will for us and the power to carry that out, so there is again the implication that we're not running things. We are empowered, but not in control. The cumulative wisdom from the pioneers of the program found early on that it's best not to make demands in prayer, but rather seek the will of a Power Greater than yourself. In this way we are bringing our heads and hearts into alignment. Even though you may have made it all the way to Step Eleven, yes, your head and heart still need additional alignment and healing.

The strength of divinity resides in all living beings. In yoga, life is seen as an expression of the Divine. We come full circle with prayer and meditation, trusting in our own intuition, so that our will aligns with the bigger picture of life. We can live in a way that honors all sentient beings.

"As you elevate your consciousness during meditation, contemplation, dreaming, and doing activities that bring forth your passion, you can sense realms outside the limitations of your physical world." -Geoffrey Jowett (2018)

The majesty of meditation is how deep the healing it facilitates. I am including a list of damages caused to the body from toxic substances from a book titled *Healing Addictive Behavior* in order to demonstrate the power meditation, inner connection, and awareness have on the whole being. If your addiction of choice does not involve ingesting chemicals, you're not quite off the hook. Acting out the addictive cycle triggers hormones that stress and depress the system, taking a similar toll on the body and brain.

Impact of Toxic Substances

The following are some general effects of toxic build-up in the body:

- *Damages brain cells and limits the brain's ability to regulate and produce neurotransmitters.*
- *Triggers an imbalance in the glandular system, compromising optimal health.*

- *Weakens the nervous system, limiting the ability to maintain self-control and mental clarity.*
- *Causes malnutrition as toxins interfere with the brain's ability to regulate nutritional needs.*

- Mukta Kaur Khalsa Ph.D. *(2014)*

I want to also make a special note about marijuana at this time. From the yogic teachings it is said that marijuana is found to create a drought like condition in the brain. It not only constricts circulation, but accumulates and stores in the brain stem, adversely affecting brain health.

Now for the good news! As mentioned, I have intentionally placed the above consequences in this chapter because meditation works directly on the areas affected and weakened by active addiction. Meditation is not only good for spiritual development, but is actually healing for the brain itself.

Benefits of Meditation

- Increased awareness
- Stress Reduction
- Increased focus and concentration
- Decreased worry and anxiety
- Increased peace, calm, and serenity
- Self-acceptance/time for self
- Increased mental balance
- Support for change and breaking old patterns
- A space to go within and work things out
- Increased awareness of the internal and external realms
- Increased discipline
- Increased connection to creative flow
- Increased spiritual connection
- Increased sense of overall well-being

Testimonial:

"I'm so honored and excited to share my experiences with Kundalini yoga. I have been taking classes for nearly two decades and fell instantly in love with the practice from my first experience. I am a survivor of abuse and a grateful woman in recovery who relies on the 12 steps in the 'Big Book' for my vital spiritual experiences. Early in my recovery, I found myself craving a deeper, more fully connected experience of my Higher Power in each of the 12 steps, especially the 11th step. In this regard, Kundalini yoga has been a game changer in my recovery as well as

my understanding of my higher power, the power of truth, the essence of yoga and how my ego operates in my mind. I've learned how to look at all aspects of life's difficulties with a beginner's mind, a quiet mind, a serene mind.

Because I'm a kinesthetic learner, it was only though Kundalini yoga that I learned HOW to maintain a constant, conscious contact with a power greater than myself. My experiences in Patty's classes can only be described as the personification of the 12 steps within my body, my heart, my soul, and my mind, not necessarily in that order. The teachings and readings help me to ward off my ego's 'Optical Rectitis' (shitty outlook on life), and remind me of the immense difference between my ego's perception and the universal reality of The Aquarian Age." -Faye V.

Bonus:

To expand your personal scope of experience, try three different spiritual practices, that are new to you, by attending classes, ceremonies, or rituals beyond your familiarity. Some ideas may be attending a church or ashram service, signing up for a meditation class (you can even try multiple styles of meditation, such as those found in the traditions of Kundalini Yoga, Buddhism, Transcendental Meditation, guided imagery, etc.), participating in a Shamanic ceremony, a sweat lodge, or a take a witch walk in the forest. The sky is the limit! Go try something new and different in the name of spiritual growth and perseverance. You may not like every new practice you try; this is just about willingness to be open. Remember, stepping out of your comfort zone strengthens your life force energy.

Yoga Recommendation:

I have chosen to include chanting as the meditation for Step Eleven in this book, as it is a vibrational expression of the Infinite. The ongoing action of prayer and meditation is supported by the seventh chakra, the connection to spirit. Mantra creates a sound vibration through the movement of the tongue and mouth which stimulates the glands in the brain. The mantra given is a chant of ecstasy describing the experience of moving from darkness to light, from ignorance to knowledge. Through immersion in the mantra, we may access the still, quiet place within the self.

Chanting Meditation

Sit in a comfortable meditation posture with the spine straight, hands on the knees in Gyan Mudra. Apply a light Root Lock to help support your spine and posture.

Chant the mantra *Wahe Guru, Wahe Guru, Wahe Guru, Wahe Jio* for 3 to 31 minutes. Chant along with the companion soundtrack to connect with the sound vibration.

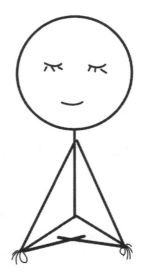

19

Step Twelve

"Having had a spiritual awakening as a result of these steps, we tried to carry this message to addicts, and to practice these principles in all our affairs."

"Being sober delivered almost everything drinking promised." - Anne Lamott (2017)

As I sit down to write on Step Twelve, I reflect upon the news I heard this morning about a woman I was in detox with in the 1980's passing away. No details were given as to the cause of death, but she had been in and out of the public eye with substance abuse problems for decades. She wasn't that much older than I, so why am I sitting here clean and sober, and why is she not? A dear friend in recovery and I spent time pondering and talking about this very question over many years. Why do some people stay in recovery to lead happy productive lives, and others struggle to get and/or stay clean, and still others end up ultimately unsuccessful? The only answer we have come up with is that we have been willing to follow direction and do the work that the program itself, and our sponsors, have suggested. That's it – willingness and action, whether we like it or not.

The actress that passed this morning shared something more than thirty years ago that has stayed with me always. She made the statement that the 12 Steps should be like taxes, in that everyone should have to work them. She had the concept that the steps are powerful tools for living a good life. What she understood on an intellectual level, enough to share with others, I went on to internalize and live, and I've never forgotten this basic premise she shared in detox – that the steps work.

So, what is a spiritual awakening mentioned in Step Twelve? In keeping it simple, when I hit bottom in my addiction I wanted to die, and after some months clean, as recovery started to take hold, I found that I wanted to live. At the time I did not even notice this subtle shift happening. When I did later recognize this new found yearning for life, it was a spiritual awakening for me. I did have an extraordinary experience early on that I kept a secret for six months. I credit this experience as the beginning of my spiritual awakening, a beginning of hope and establishing fresh new roots. As I mentioned in an earlier chapter, on my first night in treatment a roommate suggested we all pray before going to sleep, and my first reaction to the idea of prayer was total aversion. No thank you. I was happy enough knowing where I was going to sleep, eat, and shower, at least temporarily, so I certainly didn't need God.

As also mentioned, I arrived in residential treatment from a comfortable, cushy detox where I have no memory of about 6 out of 10 days, #usinggoals, and found that I was still kicking drugs and unable to sleep. After a few sleepless nights accompanied by exhaustion, irritability, and being haunted by nameless fears, I was willing to ask for help from a Power Greater than myself. Even if I left the facility, I had nowhere to go, and no one waiting for my return with open arms. My first prayer consisted of something along the lines of *"I don't believe, but I'm open."* Kind of like a dare to God to prove me wrong. As I lay in the bottom bunk with my eyes closed while my roommates slept, I put out this sincere, desperate prayer, and what I received back I took to heart. In response to my honest, unrefined request, I felt, more than heard, that it was going to be okay. I felt the words *"It's gonna be okay"* pulse through the center of my being and radiate throughout my limbs. I felt like I was floating. I was afraid if I opened my eyes the feeling would leave, so I kept them shut and remained motionless. It was a tangible experience that I clung to in the days of doubt that came ahead. I originally chalked the experience up to detoxing and no sleep, only to discount the power of what I really felt, because, as comforting as it was, it was also a little scary. I did not share this experience with a soul, until six months later on a weekend pass with a member of the fellowship I respected. She had a fun, punk rock Hollywood vibe, and openly claimed God as her center tether. She was so excited about what I shared with her and validated that, yes, this was certainly a spiritual awakening.

We actually experience many spiritual awakenings along the way. I had this kind of big one early on to draw from, but my growth from ignorance to knowledge, from darkness to light comes gradually and in increments. Yes, I did just switch to present tense because the awakening of the spirit continues; there's no end goal. In yoga we have a name for the experience of moving from darkness to light. It is *guru.* "Gu" is darkness or ignorance, and "Ru" is light or knowledge. In India a *guru* is traditionally a person who assists on the path of enlightenment, but a *guru* can be anything that sheds light where there is darkness, from a little aha moment to a profound life-changing realization. There is no right or wrong way to receive your own personal illumination or awakening.

By the time we get to Step Twelve we have reaped the benefits of working the prior eleven steps. Ideally, we have moved beyond total self-indulgence and self-centeredness in many areas of life. We are able to see that when we align our will with what we believe to be the will of our Higher Power, things work out for the better. Remember this insight comes from the heart, not the head. New-found personal freedom and contentment lead us to continue the cycle of giving and receiving, giving it away in order to keep it, and helping others as we have been helped. It's a complete circle that flows without expectation.

There is a beautiful meditation given in this book called *Kirtan Kriya* that uses ancient sounds that vibrate the cycle of life. *Sa Ta Na Ma*; infinity, life, death, and rebirth. The *mantra* reminds me of the work done in the Twelve Steps. Step Twelve brings us full circle to rebirth and we pay it forward by continuing to share the message of recovery with those in need.

As we help other people on their personal path of recovery, we revisit our past story out of the necessity of establishing common ground and internal understanding, but also so that we don't forget where we came from. Our past story does not define who we are as a person. We need not cling to it, but also not deny or obscure it. We are continually writing and editing our new story. Each day is an opportunity to build a new story, to live in the present moment of freedom from active addiction. We embrace the now, but don't forget the past so as not to slide down the slope back into the depths of a self-imposed purgatory.

In addiction we sacrifice ourselves by giving the best parts of ourselves away over and over again. However, there is an inner light that cannot be given away. It may be dimmed and diminished, but it cannot be bought, sold, taken, or extinguished. This inner light is a spark of the soul, the spirit, what I call the pulse of life, where pure love and innocence reside. Recovery awakens the light of the soul, where we once felt lost or separate, we now feel united, and this is a spiritual awakening. Once awakened we are free to share our light with others.

The principle of Step Twelve is service. In yoga it is called *seva*, or selfless service. We realize in order to help ourselves we must help others. Being of service in the program gives us the foundation to be of service beyond the rooms of recovery. This did not dawn on me until many years into recovery on a cruise to Mexico. I went on a 12 Step cruise with a friend, and our designated dinner table had us seated with people we did not previously know. One conversation led to another, and the group at the table began one-upping each other with the size and quantity of their service commitments both past and present. I sat quietly and listened until someone directed their attention to me, then asked what my current service commitments entailed. I had kids and was busy with life, plus my special needs son required me to be at multiple therapy sessions weekly, so I responded with a bit of guilt that I did not currently hold a service commitment. My friend rolled her eyes and looked at me aghast. In my defense she threw out a list of my service commitments: soccer team mom, baseball team mom, PTA, school workroom volunteer and student store coordinator, plus Girl Scouts. It turns out the basics I learned in the early days of recovery spilled over into life beyond meetings so seamlessly that I didn't even notice. I didn't even realize my volunteering with the kids was "being of service" or performing selfless *seva*.

During this time all of my service commitments, but one, were a good match. One of my responsibilities to the Girl Scout troop was to be the "cookie mom." Yes, when Girl Scout cookie season rolled around in the early spring, we had cases and cases of cookies stacked in the family room for weeks on end. I was like the connection, or the middle man, picking up a big supply of cookies to distribute in smaller quantities. I also at too much of the product. It was not a healthy or financially sound commitment for me. I share this so that you know you are allowed to make choices to be of service that support your lifestyle. You don't have to love every service commitment, but they should not be self-sabotaging.

Carrying the message of recovery and representing the 12 Step fellowship encompasses all of our interactions. How we conduct ourselves is a projection of our personal recovery and the fellowship as a whole. This holds true whether we are shopping at the mall or speaking at a meeting. It's not only about monitoring our behavior when people are watching, but actively living the steps. Are we walking like we're talking? Are we dignified, credible and reliable in all of our affairs? Step Twelve affords us the opportunity to be true to our word. The message we carry is that the steps work, and that freedom from active addiction is found through working the 12 Steps. Yoga and meditation support this process.

Testimonial:

"I came across the idea of a 'spiritual awakening' in the 12 Step program of Alcoholics Anonymous. I was spiritually awake as a child. For whatever reasons, that was dulled, and in my effort to stay awake I turned to substances and the inevitable abuse of them. I was lucky enough to realize when it wasn't working.

After several years of abstinence AA require for success, I joined Al-Anon. There I learned to apply the same steps to relationships I had with substance abusers. Eventually, I realized it worked for other situations as well.

I didn't really have a prayer or meditation practice and was not sure about the God stuff. But something was there. I faked it till I made it (it took quite a while) but I did recover that spirit. The spirit awakened, and as it stretched and yawned, I was able to hear Life calling. The direction changed. It led me to a return of a loving relationship with music, the desire to go beyond myself, to help others and the ability to joyfully (mostly) explore a spiritual practice. The 12 steps gave me the initial structure for recovery and introduced me to the very idea of an awakened spirit. They were a sturdy platform from which to leap into yoga and that awakening for now decades of sobriety. They symbiosis is extraordinary. I can thank my addiction for forcing me to recover my spirit!" - Victoria R.

Bonus:

<u>*Yogi Tea Recipe*</u>

Good for the blood, liver, nervous system, and bones. Good for colds, flu, and physical weakness.

10 ounces water
2 slices fresh ginger root (optional, but excellent!)
3 cloves
4 green cardamon pods, cracked
4 black peppercorns
½ stick cinnamon
¼ teaspoon black tea (one teabag)
½ cup milk or equivalent
Honey to taste, optional

Bring the water to a boil and add the spices. Cover and continue boiling for 10-15 minutes. Remove from heat, add black tea, and let steep for 1-2 minutes. Add honey and milk (optional), bring back to a boil and then remove from heat. Strain and serve. This recipe is for one cup, but you can make it by the gallon using the same increased proportions. -Santokh Khalsa DC (2016)

Yoga Recommendation:

The eighth chakra, or aura, supports the service work of Step Twelve. It is all encompassing. The ten body *kriya* is an amazing workout for the whole body and includes meditation at the end of the set.

"I put my hand in yours, and together we can do what we could never do alone. No longer is there a sense of hopelessness, no longer must we each depend upon our own unsteady willpower. We are all together now, reaching out our hands for power and strength greater than ours, and as we join hands, we find love and understanding beyond our wildest dreams." -OA Promise

<u>Awakening to Your Ten Bodies Kriya</u>

1. Stretch Pose. Lie down on your back. Tip the pelvis forward, then bring the feet together and raise them 6 inches from the ground, keeping the legs straight. Raise your head 6 inches and fix your eyes on the toes, which point away from you. Arms are held straight at your sides, palms facing the thighs but not touching. Hold this position for 2 to 3 minutes while performing Breath of Fire. Relax for a few seconds.

2. Nose to Knees Pose. Bend the knees to the chest, wrap the arms around them, and press them tightly into the chest. Bring the head up so that the nose comes as close to the knees as possible. Do Breath of Fire for 2 to 3 minutes. Inhale, stretch. The exhale and relax down for a few seconds before rocking back up into Easy Pose.

3. Ego Eradicator. Sitting in Easy Pose, bring the arms out to the sides, and raise them until they form a V shape. Stretch the thumbs up toward the sky. The rest of the fingers are curled onto the pads of the hands. Begin a powerful Breath of Fire while concentrating at the third-eye point. Continue for 2 to 3 minutes.

4. Spread Stretch. Spread the legs as far apart as is comfortable. Inhale and stretch up to the center. Exhale and stretch over the right leg, bringing the forehead toward the knee, and the hands to the toes if possible. Inhale up to the center again, and exhale down to the left leg, reaching the hands toward the left foot. Continue in the way for 2 to 3 minutes.

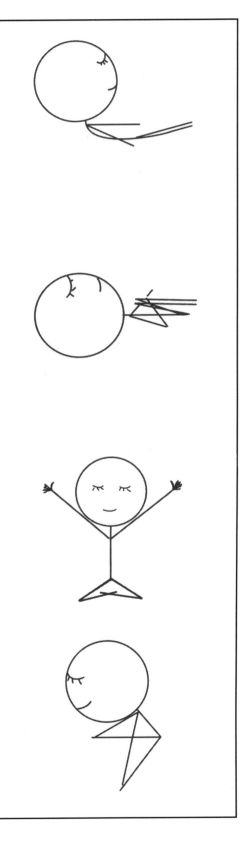

5. Center Stretch. Continue to site with the legs spread. Reach forward and grasp the toes, or, if that is not possible, hold the ankles. Inhale and stretch the head and upper body toward the floor, exhale, and sit up again. Continue for 2 to 3 minutes.

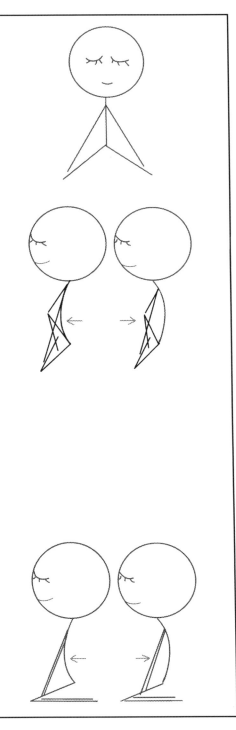

6. Lower Spinal Flex. Start by sitting on the floor with legs crossed and tucked in. Take hold of the outside of the ankle with both hands. Inhale and flex the spine forward, chest out and shoulders back. Exhale and slump the body. The shoulders curve forward, the chest caves in, and the spine is rounded. Continue in a rhythmic forward and backward manner. Focus on rocking the pelvis forward and back, as well as moving the middle and upper spine. Feel each vertebra of the spine curl and uncurl. As you continue, pick up the pace. Repeat for 2 to 3 minutes. Then inhale deeply, holding the breath. Exhale and relax the breath and the pose.

7. Camel Ride. Spinal flex sitting on the heels in Rock Pose. Place the hands flat on the thighs. Inhale and flex the spine forward with the chest out and shoulders back. Exhale, curve the chest in, and round the shoulders forward. Focus on the third-eye point as your move powerfully for 2 to 3 minutes.

8. Twists. Still sitting in Rock Pose, bring your hands up to the shoulders with the fingers in the front and the thumbs in the back. Straighten the spine and begin twisting side to side as far as you can in each direction. Keep the upper arms parallel to the ground as you swing feely from side to side. Inhale to the left and exhale to the right. Breath rhythmically and powerfully for 2 to 3 minutes.

9. Wings. Grasp the shoulders as in the previous exercise. Inhale and raise the elbows up along the sides of the head. Ideally the back of the wrists touch each other. Exhale and lower the elbows to the original position. Continue with a strong breath for 2 to 3 minutes.

10. Venus Stretch. Interlace the fingers in Venus Lock. Inhale and stretch the arms up over the head. Exhale and bring the hands back to the lap. Continue for 2 to 3 minutes.

11. Alternate and Parallel Shoulder Shrugs. Come back into Easy Pose. With the hands on the knees, make sure that the spine is straight and the neck is in line with the spine. Inhale and lift the left shoulder straight up toward the ear. Exhale as the right shoulder comes up and the left goes down. Continue with alternate shoulder shrugs for 1 minute. Then inhale and lift both shoulders up. Exhale and let the shoulders drop down. Use a powerful breath and continue up and down for 1 minute. Then inhale deeply, stretch the shoulders up, hold for a few seconds, and exhale down.

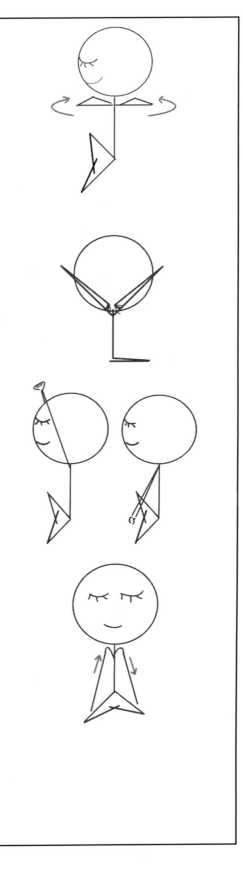

12. Head Turns. Remain in Easy Pose with the hands on the knees. Inhale and turn your head to the left. Exhale and rotate the head to the right. Continue rotating the head in this manner for 1 minute. Then reverse the breathing pattern so that you inhale as the head is turning right, exhale as it turns left. Continue for 1 minute.

13. Frog Pose. Bring the heels close together and point the toes outward. Squat down with the buttocks close to the heels, the arms between the knees, and the fingers placed on the floor about a foot in front of the feet. The upper body is as straight as possible. Inhale and straighten the legs, bringing the head close to the knees. Exhale and return to the original position. Try to keep the heels slightly off the ground the entire time. Continue for 26 to 54 repetitions, counting 1 inhalation and 1 exhalation as 1 repetition.

14. Relaxation. Deeply relax on the back for 5 to 10 minutes. Then gently wake up and prepare for meditation.

15. Laya Yoga is the recommended meditation for this kriya. Laya yoga is a form of meditation that uses rhythmic patterns or mantra and locks. The rhythm of this form easily stays within the subconscious with minimal practice. Laya yoga is very powerful and can suspend the mind in a blissful absorption with Infinity.

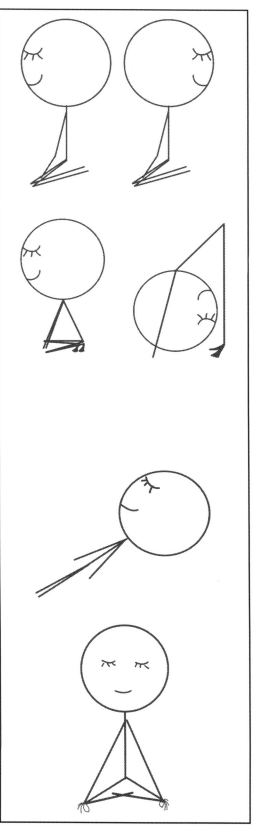

Sit in Easy Pose with the hands on the knees in Gyan Mudra (thumb and index finger touching). Chant *"Ek Ong Kar-a, Sat(a) Nam-a, Siri Wha-a, Hay Guru."* For each underlined a (pronounced like the u in bus,) in the mantra, pull the Root Lock. The focus is on the navel point pulling inward as the diaphragm is pulled up and the chest lifts. The breath will find its natural rhythm. Visualize the sound spiraling from the base of the spine to the top of the head on each repetition of the mantra. Continue for 11 minutes, increasing to a maximum of 31 minutes. *Ek Ong Kar* translates as "One Creator-Creation." *Sat Nam* means "Truth Manifested," and *Siri Wahe Guru* means "Great Indescribable Wisdom."

20

The Heart Centered Mind

Why would we want to sit on our mat in meditation to develop the neutral mind? How is it going to support a better life?

You've heard me mention the heart centered mind throughout the book. The neutral mind, the meditative mind, and the heart centered mind refer to the same aspect of the mind and can be used interchangeably. (The third functional mind, the fourth energy body, or the fourth chakra, as found in previous chapters, also reference this mind.) The developed neutral mind is the very best GPS you will ever use for your travels on earth. The neutral mind encompasses qualities of a balanced heart center; truth, clarity, and compassion. Intentionally building the neutral mind provides steady grounding and transforms the turmoil of the addictive or monkey mind. Meditation works on taming the mind and with regular practice cultivates the ability to remain observant and calm in order to take action in any given situation, rather than to unconsciously react. It clears the path for connection to truth.

What each individual has experienced in life as their own personal truths are colored by the person's emotional state at the time any given situation occurs. There are as many different truths as there are people who are present and involved in any situation. We each have "a truth," but I tend to think that "the truth" lies somewhere in the middle. The truth is neutral. In yoga this middle road is called Dharma, a righteous path wherein the individual accrues neither karmic credit or debt. Neutral action comes from the true or higher self and is in accordance with the individual's personal relationship with a Higher Power.

Neutrality circumvents the tendency for harsh judgement or angry outbursts. It allows for others to have their own experiences and opinions, and does not interpret any differences in belief or opinion as a personal attack. There is an allowance for self and for others. Without neutrality we continue to run on the same old track and see things through tired eyes. Yoga and meditation assist in this new way of life by directly working on the heart center.

When open and balanced, the fourth chakra supports an opening to feelings and compassion. The symbol for this energy center is two overlapping triangles, with a point facing both up and down. It is a space held for transition, a center without conflict. It is the true center for self-awareness and unconditional love. It is where we learn to love the self. This is where we speak from the heart. In turn, when we listen from the heart it gives the other person the feeling that they are being heard. When we drop into the heart center, we are able to be truly present.

In the space of the heart center there is a recognition that all is well no matter what. No matter what we have experienced in the past, or what comes our way in the future, at our core we may chose to remain unruffled. It is knowing that all is as it's supposed to be, in this time and place, for our life lessons. We don't have to like a situation for this to be true. We can behave badly and still circle around to come back to a steadiness within as we walk through difficult feelings. Often the most challenging of times and circumstances provide for the most growth. The bottom line is no matter what, it's going to be okay. Take a deep breath and relax. Acknowledge that you now have the ability to move through life's storms with ease and dignity. Acceptance rests in the peace of forgiveness. Deeply accepting and embracing that in the big picture all is as it should be, no matter what circumstances and emotions may be present, is what I refer to as radical neutrality.

"I sit up tall to listen to the storm.
I am stronger than the storm.
I can't sit still. I toss and turn with discomfort.
I yield, holding space with patience."

Poise and acceptance come from the heart center, not the head. If we review the three functional minds, mind being a full body phenomena, we see that the neutral mind is spacious. The negative and positive minds give input and information so that the neutral mind may make a decision based on the highest good of all involved. If we get stuck in either the positive or negative mind, we most likely form and defend an opinion, but are limited in vision and action. The ego takes over and tries to run the show. Moving through negative and positive minds to the neutral mind we find expansiveness. We have choices and options. We are not confined by opinion. Developing the neutral mind through meditation opens the door to unlimited exploration, adventure, possibility, appreciation, and acceptance.

Principles of developing the meditative mind

The Eleventh Step is the only step that uses the word meditation; however, as you can see below, the benefits reaped from meditation help to support recovery principles and the overall goal of the entire 12 Step process. The principles, or attitudes, of the meditative mind are not taught in Kundalini yoga in a succinct fashion or strict order; nor is this a complete list of attributes of the meditative mind. For the purpose of description, and demonstrating the complementary natures of recovery and yoga, I am listing yoga attributes I have chosen to highlight in an order that flows with the steps. All of these attributes reside naturally in the heart center.

1. Acceptance – There is balance in the flow of life.
2. Trust – Allowing for an alignment with the Universal Will.
3. Compassionate Detachment – Balance, surrender, loving with clarity.
4. Non-Judgement – Releasing the ego, realizing that we are all the same.
5. Gratitude – Enjoy who you are, be thankful for all lessons.
6. Awareness – Honesty, openness, connection, accountability.
7. Meditation – Trust internal messages.
8. Unconditional Love – Love of life, self, and others. A state of giving from the heart that is not reserved for only specific people.

I would like to make a further comment about the compassionate detachment mentioned above, along with the concept of surrender. Loving with detachment is surrendering attachment, dependency, and enmeshment, but it does not mean we love less. It means we know we are not in charge. For instance, I'm not beating my own heart or rotating the Earth for myself, or for you for that matter. Compassionate detachment means we love with clarity. I would like to share a little story that I heard years ago during a meditation course facilitated by Shakti Parwha Kaur Khalsa. She was talking about loving with detachment and shared a great story to explain what this actually means. I am by no means quoting her word for word, but you'll get the idea.

Imagine you are enjoying a walk through the jungle with a dear loved one, when all of the sudden your loved one steps in quicksand and begins to sink. Of course, you are going to be distraught. Loving from a place of attachment may create a panicked reaction, causing you to immediately try to save your loved one by jumping into the quicksand yourself to rescue them. What happens? You both sink. Loving from a place of compassionate-detachment supports the ability to take action from a place of truth and clarity. You can pause to assess that your loved one sinking in quicksand needs help, but rather than jumping right in to try to save them, you look around to see what would be helpful, possibly finding vines or a branch to use as a rescue tool in order to pull them out to safety. What happens? You are both out of the quicksand, alive and safe.

This story may be applied to any area of life. Jumping into the quicksand to save the sinking loved one is very similar to the attachments and dependencies found in active addiction. When we're using and trapped in the cycle of addiction, we lack the ability to see the big picture, and emotions can get the best of us, causing us to sink deeper into the dismal abyss of self-centeredness. Conversely, a clean, stable mind supports honest assessment and the ability to establish a personal program of recovery. My wish for you, is that you take some time to drop into the heart center to experience love, peace, expansion, and the freedom to engage in an amazing life.

Music

A helpful companion soundtrack titled *8 Limbs, 10 Bodies, 12 Steps: Yoga for Addiction Recovery* is available to guide you through the yoga and meditation practices found in this book. Proper pronunciation of the mantras is given, and the music provides a follow along for the practice. If music is unavailable, the meditations may be done with the focus on the breath, in most cases long, deep breathing.

The soundtrack has been recorded by yoga teacher, yoga teacher trainer, and recording artist Jap Dharam Rose. The soundtrack may be found on most popular streaming platforms.

References

Chapter One

Brand, Russell, *Recovery, Freedom from Our Addictions,* Picador by Macmillan Publishing Group, LLC. 2017

American Society of Addiction Medicine, Definition of Addiction adopted by ASAM September 2019

Gorski, Terrence T. and Miller, Merlene, *Staying Sober,* Herald Publishing House/ Independent Press 1986

Ewing, JA, *Detecting Alcoholism: The CAGE Questionaire,* JAMA 252; 1905-1907, 1984

Jellineck E.M. as found in *Loosening the Grip, A Handbook of Alcohol Information,* Times Mirror/Mosby College Publishing, 1987

Flock, Allen D., *The Addiction Model,* 1986

Addiction Angels and Answers, FB.com

Chapter Two

Bruyere, Rosalyn L., *Wheels of Light, Chakras, Auras, and the Healing Energy of the Body.* Fireside, Simon & Shuster, Inc. 1994

Bhajan, Yogi and Khalsa, Gurucharan PhD *The Aquarian Teacher: Kundalini Research Institute International Kundalini Yoga Teacher Training Level I.* Kundalini Research Institute 2003

Rose, Victoria, unpub.ms. 2022

White, Ruth, *Working With Your Chakras,* Barnes & Noble, Inc. 1993

Chapter Three

Swami Prabhavananda/Isherwood, Christopher, *How to Know God, The Yoga Aphorisms of Patanjali,* The Vedanta Society of Southern California, Vedanta Press 1953

Knox, Hansa, Yoga *Beyond the Mat, Yama and Niyama,* Yoga Matters, Yoga Alliance

Devi, Nischala Joy, *The Secret Power of Yoga,* Three Rivers Press, Random House Inc. 2007

Chopra, Deepak MD/Simon, David MD, *The Seven Spiritual Laws of Yoga,* John Wiley & Sons, Inc. 2004

Khalsa, Gurucharan PhD *The Aquarian Teacher: Kundalini Research Institute International Kundalini Yoga Teacher Training Level I,* Kundalini Research Institute 2003

Chapter Four

Khalsa, Santokh S. DC, written excerpt, unpub.ms. 2021
Khalsa, GuruMeher, *Senses of the Soul,* Kundalini Research Institute, 2013
Bhajan, Yogi and Khalsa, Gurucharan PhD *The Aquarian Teacher: Kundalini Research Institute International Kundalini Yoga Teacher Training Level I.* Kundalini Research Institute 2003
Khalsa, Siri Atma S. MD, *Waves of Healing,* Yogic Reality, Inc. 2009

Chapter Five

World Service Office, Inc., *Narcotics Anonymous,* World Service Office, Inc. 1982
Gorski, Terrence T. and Miller, Merlene, *Staying Sober,* Herald Publishing House/Independent Press 1986
World Service Office, Inc., *Living Clean,* Narcotics Anonymous World Service Office, Inc. 2012

Chapter Six

Khalsa, Gurucharan S. PhD, unpub.ms. 2022
Hooks, Bell, *All About Love,* William Morrow Paperbacks 2018
Eadie, Betty J., *Embraced by the Light,* Gold Leaf Press, 1992
Devi, Nischala Joy, *The Secret Power of Yoga,* Three Rivers Press, Random House Inc. 2007

Chapter Seven

Chopra, Deepak MD/Simon, David M.D., *The Seven Spiritual Laws of Yoga,* John Wiley & Sons, Inc. 2004
Knox, Hansa, Yoga *Beyond the Mat, Yama and Niyama,* Yoga Matters, Yoga Alliance
Khalsa, Gururattan Kaur Ph.D. https://www.yogatech.com/Guru_Rattana_Phd/Relax_and_Renew *Warm-up Set,* 1988
Bhajan, Yogi and Khalsa, Gurucharan PhD *The Aquarian Teacher: Kundalini Research Institute International Kundalini Yoga Teacher Training Level I.* Kundalini Research Institute 2003

Chapter Eight

Tolle, Eckhart, *The Power of Now,* Namaste Publishing 1999

Alcoholics Anonymous World Services, Inc., *Alcoholics Anonymous,* Alcoholics Anonymous World Services, Inc. 1939

Khalsa, Mukta Kaur Ph.D., *Meditations for Addictive Behavior,* Pettit Network Inc., Itasca Books 2008

Khalsa, Santokh DC, *Understanding Kundalini, Basic Spinal Series,* Santokh Singh Khalsa 2016

Chapter Nine

Khalsa, Shakti Parwha Kaur, *Kundalini Yoga, The Flow of Eternal Power,* First Time Capsule Books 1996

Khalsa, Gururattan Kaur Ph.D. https://www.yogatech.com/Guru_Rattana_Phd/Relax_and_Renew *Emotional Balance and Repair/Kirtan Kriya,* 1988

Chapter Ten

Bernstein, Gabrielle, *The Universe Has Your Back,* Hay House, Inc. 2016

Khalsa, Guru Prem Singh, *Divine Alignment, Kriya to Develop Navel Intelligence,* Cherdi Kala, Inc., 1969-2003

Chapter Eleven

Khalsa, GuruMeher, *Emotional Liberation,* Atmosphere Press 2021

Hay, Louise L., *Inner Wisdom, Meditations for the Heart and Soul,* Hay House, Inc. 2000

Khalsa, Shakta Kaur, *Kundalini Yoga, Kriya to Relieve Inner Anger,* Dorling Kindersley Publishing, Inc. 2001

Chapter Twelve

Michael Mejia, The Poetry of Michael, unpub.ms. 2021

Kipfer, Barbara Ann, *Natural Meditation,* Skyhorse Publishing 2018

Khalsa, Gururattan Kaur Ph.D. https://www.yogatech.com/Guru_Rattana_Phd/Relax_and_Renew *Sitali Pranayam,* 1988

Chapter Thirteen

Alcoholics Anonymous World Services, Inc., *As Bill Sees It,* Alcoholics Anonymous World Services, Inc. (1967)

Bader Ginsburg, Ruth, quote in Inc. January 12, 2019

Khalsa, Shakta Kaur, *Kundalini Yoga, Habituation Meditation,* Dorling Kindersley Publishing, Inc. 2001

Chapter Fourteen

Brand, Russell, *Recovery, Freedom from Our Addictions,* Picador by Macmillan Publishing Group, LLC. 2017

Pueblo, Yung, *Clarity & Connection,* Andrews McMeel Publishing, 2021

Amen, Daniel M.D., *Change Your Brain, Change Your Body,* Harmony Books, Random House Inc. 2010

Khalsa, Gururattan Kaur Ph.D. https://www.yogatech.com/Guru_Rattana_Phd/Relax_and_Renew *Anti-Stress Meditation,* 1988

Chapter Fifteen

Chodron, Pema, *When Things Fall Apart,* Shambhala Publications, Inc. 1997

Khalsa, Gururattan Kaur Ph.D. https://www.yogatech.com/Guru_Rattana_Phd/Relax_and_Renew *Yoga for Drug Damage, Anti-Depression and Brain Synchrony Meditation,* 1988

Chapter Sixteen

Khalsa, GuruMeher, *Senses of the Soul,* Kundalini Research Institute, 2013

Amen, Daniel M.D., *Change Your Brain, Change Your Body,* Harmony Books, Random House Inc. 2010

Chapter Seventeen

Dyer, Dr. Wayne W., *Everyday Wisdom,* Hay House, Inc. 1993

Khalsa, GuruMeher, *Senses of the Soul, Handle Yourself,* Kundalini Research Institute, 2013

Chapter Eighteen

Hawkins, David R. M.D., Ph.D., *Dissolving the Ego, Realizing the Self,* Hay House Inc. 2011

Jowett, Geoffry, *Lasting Impressions,* iUniverse 2018

Khalsa, Mukta Kaur, Ph.D., *Healing Addictive Behavior,* Pettit Network Inc., Itasca Books 2014

Rose, Jap Dharam, Recording Artist, www.japdharamrose.com, soundtracks from 2016, 2019, 2021, and 2022

Chapter Nineteen

Lamott, Anne, *Hallelujah Anyway, Rediscovering Mercy,* Riverhead Books 2017

Khalsa, Santokh DC, *Understanding Kundalini,* Santokh Singh Khalsa 2016

Khalsa, Shakta Kaur, *Kundalini Yoga, Awakening to Your Ten Bodies Kriya,* Dorling Kindersley Publishing, Inc. 2001

Rozanne S., *OA Promise*, Overeaters Anonymous, 1968

Chapter Twenty

Bhajan, Yogi and Khalsa, Gurucharan PhD *The Aquarian Teacher: Kundalini Research Institute International Kundalini Yoga Teacher Training Level I.* Kundalini Research Institute 2003

Resources

Alcoholics Anonymous World Service Office

Khalsa, Guru Prem, *Divine Alignment*
www.divinealignment.com

Khalsa, GuruMeher, *Senses of the Soul and Emotional Liberation*
www.sensesofthesoul.com

Khalsa, Gururattan Kaur, PdD, *Relax and Renew*
www.yogatech.com

Khalsa, Santokh DC, *Understanding Kundalini*
www.khalsachiropracticpasadena.com

Khalsa, Shakta Kaur, *Kundalini Yoga*
www.childrensyoga.com

KRI -Kundalini Research Institute
www.kundaliniresearchinstitute.org

Narcotics Anonymous World Service Office